Coming Home

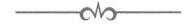

Coming Home

How Midwives Changed Birth

Wendy Kline

OXFORD
UNIVERSITY PRESS

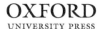

OXFORD

UNIVERSITY PRESS

Oxford University Press is a department of the University of Oxford. It furthers
the University's objective of excellence in research, scholarship, and education
by publishing worldwide. Oxford is a registered trade mark of Oxford University
Press in the UK and certain other countries.

Published in the United States of America by Oxford University Press
198 Madison Avenue, New York, NY 10016, United States of America.

© Oxford University Press 2019

Portions appear in the following works:
"Back to Bed: From Hospital to Home Obstetrics in the City of Chicago," *Journal of the
History of Medicine and Allied Sciences*, Vol. 73 (1), pp. 29–51, January 2018.
"The Little Manual That Started a Revolution: How Hippie Midwifery Became Mainstream,"
in David Kaiser and Patrick McCray, eds., *Groovy Science: The Countercultural Embrace of
Science and Technology over the Long 1970s* (Chicago: University of Chicago Press, 2016).
"Communicating a New Consciousness: Countercultural Print and the Home Birth Movement
in the 1970s," *Bulletin of the History of Medicine*, Vol. 89 (Fall 2015).

Library of Congress Cataloging-in-Publication Data
Names: Kline, Wendy, 1968– author.
Title: Coming home : how midwives changed birth / Wendy Kline.
Description: New York : Oxford University Press, [2019] | Includes
bibliographical references and index.
Identifiers: LCCN 2018027018 (print) | LCCN 2018046609 (ebook) |
ISBN 9780190232528 (Updf) | ISBN 9780190232535 (Epub) |
ISBN 9780190232511 (hardcover : alk. paper)
Subjects: LCSH: Midwifery—United States—History. |
Midwives—United States. | Childbirth—United States.
Classification: LCC RG950 (ebook) | LCC RG950.K57 2019 (print) |
DDC 618.200973—dc23
LC record available at https://lccn.loc.gov/2018027018

1 3 5 7 9 8 6 4 2

Printed by Sheridan Books, Inc., United States of America

For Brigette

CONTENTS

ACKNOWLEDGMENTS

Researching and writing this book has been an incredible adventure. My children were both born in the hospital, and I never imagined I would be drawn to the topic of home birth when I became a historian. And yet, as I hope the following pages demonstrate, the history of home birth is both fascinating and important. The sources and stories that I discovered along the way kept me reading, researching, asking questions, and hungry for more.

None of this would have happened without support from several institutions. Through their generosity, I was able to attend multiple midwifery conferences, take a weeklong midwifery assistant workshop on The Farm in Summertown, Tennessee, and travel all over the globe to meet with midwives, activists, consumers, and doctors to learn more about the subject. A fellowship in the history of medicine from the American College of Obstetricians and Gynecologists enabled me to spend a month in Washington, D.C., working in the ACOG library as well as the National Library of Medicine, which houses the papers of the American College of Nurse-Midwives. The Sophia Smith Collection at Smith College provided funding for me to research the papers of the Midwives Alliance of North America, along with the personal papers of Carol Leonard. Numerous grants from the University of Cincinnati, including a yearlong fellowship and summer support from the Charles Phelps Taft Center, gave me the much-needed time to research and write. I also received support from Purdue University's College of Liberal Arts, including several travel grants and an Enhancing Research in the Humanities and the Arts summer support grant.

This is a book about personal stories, and it could not have been written without the trust and generosity of many people. The following individuals donated their time, sharing memories, experiences, and oftentimes personal documents that helped to shape this book, taking me everywhere from Manhattan to Tenerife to Bali: Diana Altman, Suzanne Arms, Alice Bailes, Rahima Baldwin, Linda Bennett, Kate Bowland, Erica Chapin, Beth Coyote, Gene Declerq, Andrea Dixon, Karen Ehrlich, Jan Epstein,

Mary Fjerstad, Kay Furey, Ina May Gaskin, Faith Gibson, Cara Gillette, Patsy Harman, Esther Herman, Pamela Hunt, Rhona Jacobs, Roberta Kvenild, Karen Laing, Raven Lang, Carol Leonard, Robin Lim, Judy Luce, Marian Tompson, Elan McAllister, Marion McCartney, Shafia Monroe, Jo Anne Myers-Ciecko, Suzy Myers, Jane Reyes, Joanne Santana, Paul Schattauer, Phil Schweitzer, Mary Sommers, Phyllis Stein, Fran Ventre, Eva Wax, Siobhan Whalen, and Rachel Dolan Wickersham. I can't thank you enough—this is your history and I am honored to be entrusted with it. It was impossible to include as much as I wanted to, but I hope this is just the beginning and that there will be many more histories to follow.

Writing can be a lonely and intimidating process, but I found myself surrounded by support. Three archivists in particular have been extremely helpful in tracking down important materials and finding good images for the book: Debra Scarbrough of the American College of Obstetricians and Gynecologists; Susan Sacharski of the Northwestern Memorial Hospital Archives; and Stephanie Schmitz of the Purdue University Archives and Special Collections.

Thank you also to the following colleagues who generously read through chapter drafts and provided extremely helpful feedback: Evie Blackwood, Katie Brownell, Carrie Janney, Becky Kluchin, Judy Leavitt, Paula Michaels, Yvonne Pitts, Randy Roberts, Margaret Tillman, Dominique Tobbell, and Jackie Wolf. And a very special thank you to my editor, Susan Ferber, who did an incredible job of making this a more readable book, along with the two anonymous reviewers. My good friend and historian Tiffany Wayne deserves huge credit for producing the book's index—third time in a row! As always, I received excellent feedback from friends and colleagues at the annual meetings of the American Association for the History of Medicine, where I presented much of this material. Special thanks to the regulars who are always supportive: Rima Apple, David Barnes, Charlotte Borst, Winifred Connerton, Pat D'Antonio, Jackie Duffin, Erika Dyck, Julie Fairman, Janet Golden, Jeremy Greene, David Herzberg, Margaret Humphreys, Judy Houck, Laura Kelly, Baron Lerner, Anne Kviem Lie, Beth Linker, Jessica Martucci, Rich McKay, Susan Reverby, Naomi Rogers, Dominique Tobbell, Nancy Tomes, Keith Wailoo, Liz Watkins, Jackie Wolf, and John Warner. And Becky Kluchin, as always, you've kept me going not just at conferences but through our weekly check-ins.

Over the years of working on this book I left one history department and joined another. Many thanks to my former colleagues at the University of Cincinnati who shared support and feedback, especially Isaac Campos, Erika Gasser, Stephen Porter, Kate Sorrels, and David Stradling. Thank you to my former graduate students, Evan Hart, Brittany Cowgill, Alyssa McClanahan, and Anne Steinert for your invaluable insights, and for your help on this project. At Purdue University, I've been blessed with terrific colleagues who have taught me so much over the past few years. Special thanks to David Atkinson, Jean Beaman, Evie Blackwood, Katie Brownell, Fritz Davis, Will Gray, Ellen Gruenbaum, Cole Jones, Carrie Janney, Brian Leung, Silvia Mitchell, Yvonne Pitts, Randy Roberts, Margaret Tillman, Sharra Vostral, Whitney Walton, and Laurel Weldon.

I'm very grateful to friends and family members who have been patient and supportive during this long process, especially Tara Greene (who took the author photograph), Susan Shorr, Laurie Hermundson, Sylvia Sellers-Garcia, Jennifer Lloyd, Cinda Macrory, Chandrika Kasturi, Diana Hardy, Tamara and Tony Hazbun, Kate and Neil Mascarenhas, Regan Bailey, Libby Richards, Jason Brownell, Nick Palmer, Tiffany Wayne, Rachel Young, Susie McPeck, Nancy Kline, Peter Kline, Syril Kline, Maureen Kline, Stephanie Desjardins, and Barbara Gardner. Thank you to Stefan Paula for all of your incredible support and encouragement and for being a terrific father to Emily and Max. When I began this project Emily was only eight years old and Max was twelve. They've grown up with this project and know more about midwives and home birth than they ever wanted to—thanks, guys. A special thank you to little Ben, who provided me with solitude and a clean desk to write the final words of this book. And finally, thank you to Brigette, for believing in me. It has made all the difference.

Coming Home

᠎

Introduction

From Hospital to Home

O n December 8, 2009, Brazilian supermodel Giselle Bundchen and Patriots quarterback Tom Brady welcomed their son Rein into the world. Unlike the majority of babies born in the United States, Rein's first view was not of a hospital delivery room, but of his parents' Beacon Hill penthouse overlooking the Charles River in Boston. Why was he born at home? "I wanted to experience the transformation," Bundchen explained in an interview for *Vogue.* "It was the most amazing experience of my life, feeling him come through my body. And once he was born, I never felt so empowered as looking at him and thinking, Oh, my God, we did it together!" If she had given birth in a hospital, either domestically or in her home country of Brazil, her chances for a vaginal birth would have been greatly reduced. American cesarean section rates had increased by 46 percent during the first decade of the twenty-first century, up to 32 percent, while in Brazil, rates had risen to 55 percent.[1]

Bundchen joined a number of celebrities—Demi Moore, Meryl Streep, Julianne Moore, Jennifer Connelly, and Cindy Crawford, to name a few— who have opted for a home birth and generated flashy headlines about the birthing practice.[2] "Gisele Bundchen Makes Water Birth Sexy," announced ABC News. Because hers was a water birth, reporters quipped that though the practice wasn't new, Bundchen's delivery "brings a lot more splash to the concept."[3]

The idea that home birth could be sexy, splashy, or even desirable shocked many Americans, who have little knowledge of the history of midwifery or home birth. If they know anything at all, it was probably from having watched *The Business of Being Born*, a 2008 documentary produced by and featuring another celebrity, Ricki Lake. Bundchen and many others attribute their decisions to give birth at home to that film. Attended by a home birth midwife, Lake had her son in her bathtub and included footage of the birth in the documentary. The film quickly jumped to #28 on the Netflix top fifty streamed films. One midwife with a home birth practice noted that nine out of every ten of her home birth clients have come to her as a result of Lake's documentary.[4] Medical anthropologist Robbie Davis-Floyd, featured in the film, told *Associated Press* that although home birth was a "hippie, countercultural thing in the 1970s," midwives have become "increasingly sophisticated, [and] so has their clientele."[5]

The reasons for the recent trend are, of course, far more complex than a single film and are part of the longer history of midwifery and home birth in the United States. In colonial America, childbirth practices resembled those of England, where it was entirely a female affair.[6] Beginning in the 1760s, American physicians developed an interest in normal obstetrics and gradually replaced female midwives.[7] William Shippen, for example, provided a series of lectures on midwifery to male physicians after returning from medical training in England in 1762. He opened a practice of midwifery in Philadelphia and "became a favorite of Philadelphia's established families."[8] Others followed suit, expanding their practices to include laboring women. Women who opted for this new "man midwife"—and could afford him—believed him to possess a skill lacking in the female midwife.[9] Men had far greater access to medical education than did women and were more likely to use obstetrical tools, such as forceps or anesthesia. Midwife Martha Ballard revealed her frustration when a new male physician was called in to help at a birth. "At Mr. Sewall's," she wrote in her diary on October 10, 1794. "They were intimidated & Calld Dr. Page who gave my patient 20 drops of Laudanum which put her into such a stupor her pains (which were regular & promising) in a manner stopt till near night when she pukt & they returned & shee delivered at 7 hour Evening of a Son, her first Born."[10] She believed that Dr. Page was more of a nuisance than a help. "It is probable that physicians' techniques created new problems for birthing women and actually increased the dangers of childbirth," notes historian Judith Leavitt.[11]

By the early twentieth century, physician-attended birth had become the norm. In 1900, midwives participated in approximately half of all births; by 1930, that number was down to 15 percent. "Midwifery was left to become a curious historical artifact with a sometimes dubious reputation," explains one historian of childbirth.[12] Within the decade, hospital replaced home as the primary location of childbirth. Thus both the attendant and the place of birth shifted in the early twentieth century and ushered in a new era of medicalized birth.

Not everyone viewed the new medical model of childbirth as a sign of progress. Patricia Cloyd Carter, who delivered six of her nine children at home without any assistance, ranted against the practice of hospital births. "Already in some pain as the average parturient is at the end of dilation, being held tied down, slapped, shaken by the shoulders, ordered 'Stop bearing down' in tones you wouldn't use to a dog. Imagine yourself struggling against not one, but several nurses, as there always seem plenty on hand for this sadism, no matter how short they are of nurses to change a baby's wet diaper. (Six ganged me.)"[13] Carter wrote and self-published what might be the first "how to" home birth manual in 1957.[14] "EXTRA!! NEWBORN IN PRESENCE OF FATHER WITH NO PROTECTIVE GLASS BETWEEN THEM," she quips in a caption beneath a photo of her with her ten-minute-old son and husband. Her husband's clothes were not sterile, she continued. "They are merely his pajamas, and Mrs. Carter still has on the dress she wore when he was born. [Baby] Douglass does not appear to be alarmed at this, or at the absence of masks."[15]

Carter was one of a growing number of consumers dismayed by the emotional and physical toll of medicalized childbirth. "What should have been the most exalting and exulting of experiences was riddled with horrors at a big inner-city hospital where I felt like I was going to the Bastille, not to be seen again," reflected one woman. "The delivery room was an immensely bloody spectacle in what seemed at the time like a butcher shop where everyone was wearing rubber gloves and I was in the middle like a trussed-up turkey."[16] The new American midwife, "not the muslin-skirted, mule-riding, frontier type, but a medically competent, highly skilled professional," would help to reform childbirth.[17] In 1977, the founders of the consumer organization NAPSAC (National Association of Parents and Professionals for Safe Alternatives in Childbirth) predicted at a conference that "childbirth of the future will not primarily be in hospitals, but in the home, and the primary health professional for most women will not be the physician, but the midwife." Even the title of the conference and resulting book, *21st Century Obstetrics Now!* hinted at the optimism that the mainstreaming of home birth lay just around the corner.

They were wrong, of course. And yet, in 1977, their optimism seemed justified. Things had come a long way; a short time before, both midwifery and home birth appeared destined for extinction. As recently as 1970, the percentage of hospital births reached an all-time high of 99.4 percent. Then, seemingly out of nowhere, a host of new alternative organizations, publications, and conferences appeared, signaling a very different demographic trend. By 1977, the percentage of out-of-hospital births had more than doubled. A quiet revolution spread across cities and suburbs, towns and farms, as consumers challenged legal, institutional, and medical protocols by choosing unlicensed midwives to catch their babies at home. *Coming Home* narrates the ideas, values, and experiences that led to this quiet revolution and its long-term consequences for birth, medicine, and American culture.

Who were these self-proclaimed midwives, and how did they learn their trade? Because the United States had virtually eliminated midwifery in most areas by the mid-twentieth century, many of them had little knowledge of or exposure to the historic practice. Instead they learned their craft from obstetrical texts, trial and error, and sometimes instruction from the few remaining home birth physicians. While their constituents were primarily drawn from the educated white middle class, their model of care (which ultimately drew on the wisdom and practice of a more diverse, global pool of midwives) had the potential to transform birth practices for all women, both in and out of the hospital.

This is a story not just about midwives, but also about birthplace. By the 1970s, a significant number of white middle-class parents began opting out of the standardized medicated hospital birth. By doing so, they re-cast home birth as a legitimate choice for those seeking more control over the birthing process, rather than as a low-cost alternative for the poor or geographically isolated, as it had been before. This transition indicated a shift in the demographics of home birth advocates, who from their eco-nomically privileged position viewed the hospital setting as inferior to the home. "Most home deliveries used to result from economic need or lack of hospital facilities," noted Dr. William C. Scott in 1980. "The kind of family that today is demanding a different type of delivery is a far cry from the economically and socially deprived patients who used to be cared for by lay midwives."[18]

Many women who chose home birth linked their decision to power dy-namics. "It had something to do with control, power, and authority," so-ciologist Barbara Katz Rothman explained of her own decision to choose home birth in the early 1970s. "At home, I would have them; in the hos-pital they were handed over to the institution."[19] Three members of the Boston Women's Health Book Collective, which had authored *Our Bodies, Ourselves*, had given birth at home. As Judy Norsigian and Jane Pincus wrote on behalf of the collective, "several of us . . . know firsthand the joys and comforts of having our babies in a warm, familiar setting surrounded by loved ones and skilled, sensitive birth attendants."[20] While Katz Rothman focused on the power of place, Norsigian and Pincus emphasized the com-forts of home. Warm and familiar, it was, in essence, womblike.

Other home birth advocates, however, emphasized home as an idea rather than an actual physical place. "Home birth is not really about where a baby is born but is, rather, a metaphor for an attitude," wrote Diana Altman, co-founder of Birth Day, a home birth organization in Boston in the 1970s. She believed that it spoke to a woman's willingness to take responsibility for the important events of her life. Furthermore, it was an attitude that acknowledged "that the birth process is, usually, just as it should be, a perfect expression of a woman's sexuality." To Altman and many others, home birth was about privacy and intimacy, not about familiarity or comfort.

Their stories need to be told. Over thirty years ago, historian Judith Walzer Leavitt published her groundbreaking study, *Brought to Bed: Childbearing in America, 1750–1950,* which established the legitimacy and value of historicizing childbirth and inspired a new generation of scholars to research the intersections between reproduction, medicine, and feminism, emphasizing women's active roles in changing birth practices. Other works have detailed important aspects of postwar birth practices such as the growing interest in the Lamaze method, concerns about the effects of drugs used in hospital deliveries, the rise of cesarean sections, and the role of fathers in reforming maternity ward protocols, but they have not examined how alternative practitioners and the consumers who sought them out challenged obstetric practice and assumptions about birth, and how organized medicine responded.[21]

In reconstructing this history, this book draws on the papers of midwives, educators, and activists; organizations of midwives and obstetricians; and interviews with some of the key figures in the home birth movement. To have access to both archival papers and their original owners is a historian's dream. Frequently, the presence of a historical document triggered a memory or inspired a fruitful conversation. Sometimes, it was the reverse; a memory would result in a discovery of an old document stored in a midwife's attic or garage. Interviewing midwives in groups reunited for the first time in years enabled individuals to spark collective memories and to assess challenges and successes together from hindsight. And witnessing them in action—whether in their offices or at professional conferences—served as a reminder that these women were practitioners as well as revolutionaries.

This book moves from mid-century Chicago to suburban Washington D.C. to the more countercultural West Coast. At the beginning of this movement, it was very much a local phenomenon, with very little awareness that other communities were experiencing similar trends. Each chapter is situated in a different geographic locale, but also tackles a different issue that addresses why a small though increasing number of women chose home over hospital in the late twentieth century, and how a growing number of women decided to organize and professionalize around the issue of home birth. This book challenges six basic assumptions surrounding birth and society in the late twentieth century: the process of medicalization, the meaning of counterculture, the psychology of birth, the legality of licensure, and the processes of midwifery professionalization and education. While the book's focus is on a specific type of birthplace and birth practitioner, it paints a broader picture of reproductive revolution and reform in modern America.

The story begins in Chicago, where two movements converged that lay the groundwork for a burgeoning home birth movement. Chapter 1, "Back to Bed: From Hospital to Home Obstetrics in the City of Chicago," analyzes the home obstetrics training practiced at the Chicago Maternity Center alongside the emergence of what would become an international breastfeeding organization, La Leche League (LLL). Interest in breastfeeding also galvanized a movement of primarily white middle-class women in suburban Washington D.C. to challenge hospital birth practices. Chapter 2, "Middle-Class Midwifery: Transforming Birth Practices in Suburban Washington D.C.," investigates the individuals and organizations that began to promote home birth in the 1970s. Many of the D.C. area women attribute their "calling" to midwifery at least in part to their experiences as mothers, LLL leaders, and childbirth educators. When they opted to take the further step of becoming midwives, they enabled the transition of home birth as a practice primarily supervised by doctors to one facilitated by midwives. On the West Coast, a 1970s home birth was far more likely to occur in a teepee or a commune than a ranch house, as in suburban Maryland. Chapter 3, "Psychedelic Birth: The Emergence of the Hippie Midwife," focuses on the spirituality and psychology of birth more frequently espoused on the West Coast. In this context, childbirth became a catalyst to spiritual transcendence. Chapter 4, "The Bowland Bust: Medicine and the Law in Santa Cruz, California," traces the role of the hippie midwife from the perspective of a legal case. In the spring of 1974, three women were arrested in an undercover sting operation in Santa Cruz and charged with practicing medicine without a license for their involvement in out-of-hospital births coordinated by the Santa Cruz Birth Center. The birth center bust and the players involved showcase the potential for collaboration—between midwives and doctors, feminists and back-to-the-landers, politicians and activists—as well as the obstacles that ultimately prevented them from doing so.

The final two chapters address the politics of direct-entry midwifery professionalization and education. What had previously been "isolated pockets of consciousness," as midwife Kate Bowland described the relatively small groups of midwives practicing underground, had become by the late 1970s a burgeoning profession. This was facilitated by efforts to create a national organization to represent lay midwives. Chapter 5, "From El Paso to Lexington: The Formation of the Midwives Alliance of North America," closely tracks the push to organize, beginning with the first international conference of practicing midwives in El Paso in 1978 and ending with the formation of MANA.

One of the biggest hurdles to professionalizing non-nurse midwifery was the lack of any standardized training opportunities in the United States. Historically, midwives had learned their trade by apprenticing with more experienced members of their community. By the late twentieth century, however, the home birth trend triggered a regulatory backlash in many states, resulting in new and more restrictive licensure laws requiring education and certification. The final chapter, "From Professionalization to Education: The Creation of the Seattle Midwifery School," traces the evolution of the first and arguably the most successful fully accredited direct-entry midwifery program recognized by the U.S. Department of Education.

The status of midwifery care in the United States has improved in the twenty-first century, but it lags well behind those of other countries. In the United Kingdom, midwives deliver half of all babies, while in the United States midwives attend approximately 10 percent of all births. The vast majority of the 15,000 midwives in the United States are Certified Nurse-Midwives (CNMs) practicing in hospitals. The rest are Certified Midwives (CMs) or Certified Professional Midwives (CPMs), both "direct-entry" midwives without nursing credentials. While CNMs can practice legally in all fifty states, CPMs can obtain licensure in thirty states and CMs in five. CPMs work primarily in home and birth center settings and "typically cannot obtain hospital practice privileges and often have difficulty establishing reliable systems for referral and collaborative care." "It's very confusing," admits a former president of the American College of Nurse-Midwives. "The title 'midwife' has multiple meanings," making it more challenging to promote the profession.

In 2014, the medical journal *Lancet* published a series of four articles and five comments on the status of midwifery worldwide. "Midwifery is commonly misunderstood," explained the editors. They were intent on correcting that misunderstanding. Increasing collaboration by integrating midwives into health care systems could potentially prevent more than 80 percent of maternal and infant deaths, they found. "Midwifery therefore has a pivotal, yet widely neglected, part to play in accelerating progress to end preventable mortality of women and children."[22]

That recommendation does not sit well with many Americans, despite the fact that maternal mortality is on the rise, and access to affordable healthcare is shrinking. Many of them continue to see the midwife as either an ancient relic or an uneducated buffoon, unaware of her rich history and present practice in hospitals, birth centers, and homes. Midwifery organizations are challenging this by creating public education campaigns about their important role in maternity care. "Is it really such a radical idea that midwives take over low risk maternity care?" MANA president Vicki Hedley asked in May of 2018. "What is the status quo in this country? It is a system with little regard for women's bodies and no respect for their intelligence," she adds. "Let's set the table, let's invite those who truly want to serve birthing people, let's find a way to define midwifery in this country that is autonomous, inclusive, respectful, and sacred."[23]

In order to do this, we need to invest not only in midwifery's future, but also its past. We must explore the varied pathways and particular places, including the home, which shaped the profession. This book is intended to further that story.

CHAPTER 1

Back to Bed

From Hospital to Home Obstetrics
in the City of Chicago

From the time she was born, Kay Furey believes, she was a midwife in training. The oldest of thirteen children, she accompanied her mother to all of her prenatal visits in the 1940s and 1950s on the South side of Chicago. Like many families living in that neighborhood, Kay's family had emigrated from eastern Europe, where her grandmother had practiced as a midwife in Ukraine. As an adult, Kay would deliver over a thousand babies, including her nine sisters' children, at home. "You have your babies at home. That's what you do," she explained.[1] Home birth seemed quite normal to her, despite the fact that it had become a rarity in the United States. Most pregnant women were not opting to give birth at home in the mid-twentieth century, particularly in large cities.

Chicago was different. What happened in this Midwestern city lay the groundwork for a burgeoning home birth movement, as well as increasing interest in midwifery, across the United States over the coming decades. Kay Furey was one of tens of thousands of women in Chicago who bucked the trend of a hospital birth and a bottle-fed baby. She was able to give birth at home, breastfeed her children, and eventually become a home birth midwife because of two very different local establishments: the Chicago Maternity Center and La Leche League.[2]

Most would not view the Chicago Maternity Center (CMC) founder Dr. Joseph DeLee, known as the "father of American obstetrics," as a proponent of home birth, since he is credited as the man responsible for moving birth from home to hospital.[3] Nor would most assume that Marian Tompson or the other Roman Catholic founding mothers of the breastfeeding support group La Leche League (LLL) would support the fairly radical notion that women had the right to choose how and where to give birth. But an analysis of these founders' motivations reveals a unique confluence of ideas and opportunities that shaped local birth practices both for the inner-city poor and the suburban middle class.

A close examination of the rise of and reaction to modern obstetrics in twentieth-century Chicago challenges the oppositional model between home delivery and modern obstetrics that has been entrenched in American culture. Home birth continued to flourish in Chicago long after it had largely disappeared from other cities and before it returned as a countercultural practice. The underlying reasons for its sustenance varied dramatically and depended on class and context. Under DeLee and the CMC, home birth provided essential training for obstetrical students, while under Tompson and the LLL, it enabled mothers to breastfeed and bond with their babies. Taken together, these two stories reveal the complex origins of what would become a contested yet increasingly popular practice decades later.

TEACHING OBSTETRICS: JOSEPH DELEE AND THE CHICAGO MATERNITY CENTER

Chicago was home to one of the most influential obstetricians during the first half of the twentieth century. Dr. Joseph DeLee opened Chicago's first maternity dispensary in 1895 and the Chicago Lying-In Hospital in 1899. His obstetrics textbook, *The Principles and Practice of Obstetrics*, was first published in 1913 and went through thirteen editions.[4] He was featured on the cover of *Time* magazine in 1936 and referred to as "the best obstetrician in the U.S."[5]

DeLee's primary goal was to elevate the specialty of obstetrics within the American medical field. As head of the department of obstetrics at Northwestern University, and later Chair of the Department of Obstetrics and Gynecology at the University of Chicago, he played a major role in shaping and legitimizing the field. His biographer referred to DeLee as a "Crusading Obstetrician," who selflessly raised the status of childbirth to a "scientific procedure."[6] DeLee blamed two groups of practitioners for the high rates of infant and maternal mortality in the early twentieth century: midwives and poorly trained general practitioners. "The usual midwife of today," DeLee testified in court in 1916, "is a very ignorant, unconscientious and really impossible person."[7] General practitioners who delivered babies lacked adequate training because medical schools offered few opportunities for clinical experience. Most students learned obstetrics only through lecture and practice on a manikin.[8]

DeLee knew about the lack of training from his own experience as a medical student at Chicago Medical College (later Northwestern University Medical School). "We students had very good obstetric lectures and work on the manikin, but obstetric material was woefully lacking," he told doctors at a hospital banquet in 1938. "We would cajole some poor soul whom we picked up in the pediatric dispensary to let [their instructor] deliver her before the class. We passed the hat; each student chipped in fifty cents."[9] Possibilities for witnessing or participating in a home delivery were even more limited. Students were not typically welcomed as apprentices in private obstetric practice, which meant that their only opportunities came from hospital or Dispensary patients (usually the poor).[10] "Occasionally a student could wangle an old motherly woman to allow him to deliver her at home, and usually when he did so the woman would tell him to conduct the labor, which she knew more about than he did," DeLee recalled. The school forbade this practice after a lawsuit was filed against it by a husband whose laboring wife died of infection.[11] DeLee's biographer, Morris Fishbein, also a Chicago physician, noted in his own autobiography that while a student at Rush Medical College in Chicago he "received better instruction" from a poor Irish woman whose eighth birth he attended than he ever had in any classroom: "She was thoroughly familiar with every step of the process."[12]

Neither Fishbein nor DeLee viewed this state of affairs as a positive endorsement for the state of obstetrics in the early twentieth century. The real expert should not be the mother, but the obstetrician. As a medical student, DeLee had the opportunity to study home obstetric services in Berlin, Paris, Vienna, and New York City. The founders of the New York Dispensary warmly welcomed DeLee, who "learned much from their experience and was greatly inspired and encouraged by their success."[13] He set out to "remedy the same evils" by creating a similar clinic for Chicago's needy, and on February 14, 1895, opened the Maxwell Street Dispensary.[14] It was initially housed in a four-room apartment on the corner of Maxwell Street and Newberry Avenue, a densely packed immigrant neighborhood DeLee believed was "needing the institution most."[15] According to DeLee, patient applications quickly came from multiple locations, including charitable associations such as the Visiting Nurses' Association and Hull House.[16] The following year, the clinic moved across the street to larger quarters, where it remained until 1973.[17] All deliveries took place at home. For cases requiring surgery, DeLee opened a small, fifteen-bed hospital in 1899.

It was the smaller hospital—not the home birth–oriented Dispensary— that interested the University of Chicago in the 1920s. DeLee accepted a position at the university and a new, modern version of his hospital was constructed on the university's Midway campus.[18] Unfortunately, this move jeopardized the Maxwell Street Dispensary. Much to DeLee's dismay, the new hospital board of directors voted to close it in 1931, anticipating the nationwide shift in childbirth patterns from home to hospital.

DeLee called the move a "calamitous action" and set to work raising funds to keep the Dispensary open.[19] In the process of fundraising, he articulated a rationale for home birth that would far outlast him. "We can care for five times as many women for the same expenditure of money" as would be spent for a hospital delivery, "and we actually reduce the number of mothers dying in childbirth and thus the amount of indigency in the community," DeLee wrote.[20] Home births were, simply put, cheaper and safer than hospital births. Why eliminate the more cost-effective option?

Many advocates came forward in support of saving the Maxwell Street Dispensary. "It has stood out all of these years as a beacon [of] light for so many of our poor mothers, that we do not know how to plan without it," wrote one nurse. These patients were women who could not afford the cost or the travel expenses to the University of Chicago Hospital. "A trip to the moon is just about as easily accomplished as a trip to the new hospital on the Midway by most of them."[21]

For many expectant mothers, cost and distance were two of the factors they faced; changing demographics and racial discrimination also impacted their birthing options. Between 1920 and 1930, the black population in Chicago increased by over 113 percent (up to 233,903). The 1930 census documented a "rigidly segregated ghetto,"[22] as over two-thirds of black Chicagoans lived in separate neighborhoods from white Chicagoans.[23] African-American women in labor were routinely sent to Cook County Hospital, which would admit patients regardless of race or ability to pay. Even before the Depression, most locals viewed Cook County as "the place of last resort,"[24] a reputation that clung to the hospital for decades. "My first child was born at Cook County Hospital," stated an African-American mother in 1972. "They don't treat you nice like they do at home."[25] This was one more reason, many believed, to opt for a home delivery.

For DeLee, a woman's right to choose where to give birth was not the main rationale for providing home obstetrics. Medical training was. Delivering babies at home offered the opportunity to advance obstetrical knowledge by providing hands-on training in an important setting. "We can teach students and doctors how to do good routine obstetrics in the poorest hovel," DeLee wrote. Despite his desire to move childbirth to the hospital, he believed that the best learning opportunities took place in the "adverse conditions of the home" rather than in a "finely equipped hospital." The challenge, he believed, was how to expose doctors and students to enough complicated cases to develop their obstetrical skills. In the future, he hoped, all births would take place in the hospital. But in order to ensure that shift, obstetrical training needed to incorporate far more than the one or two hospital deliveries that most medical students had the opportunity to witness. They needed to learn how to treat complicated cases "under the most unfavorable conditions," where access to hospital technology might not be available. "Closing the Dispensary there will deprive us of this valuable part of our curriculum of instruction . . . and also reduce our supply of pathologic material for research."[26]

Through successful fundraising and eventual affiliation with Northwestern University, the Dispensary's practice of home obstetrics continued under the name of the Chicago Maternity Center (CMC). While the location was the same, near Jane Addams' Hull House, the board of directors and medical staff were completely new. DeLee hired Dr. Beatrice Tucker as medical director in 1932. A total of 3,386 babies were born at home with the assistance of CMC staff during her first year.[27]

Tucker had just finished her residency in obstetrics at the University of Chicago when DeLee approached her about becoming the director of the new CMC. At six feet tall, she struck an imposing figure and was quick to challenge DeLee or anyone else who treated her any differently than her male colleagues. "He did try to get a male first, and he couldn't get anybody down there because they were interested in making money," Tucker remembered. "I said that I wanted to make money, too." But she decided she liked home obstetrics, which she had already done as part of her residency under the direction of DeLee. "Dr. DeLee believed in home delivery. He really did." He stressed how much more students could learn from a home delivery, where the students sat with the patient during the entire labor, rather than in the hospital, where they worked in shifts. "You learn all the physiology of childbirth and you have to know that and know it well before you can really apply your obstetrical knowledge and manage and deliver a baby properly."[28] So she agreed to run the Maternity Center, where she proceeded to spend forty-one years training medical students and residents.

Tucker was the CMC's ideal missionary. In annual reports she stressed how the CMC benefited both poor families and the field of obstetrics. "Caring for poor women in their homes has outstanding social values," she wrote in 1933. It helped to keep families together and improved birth outcomes. While the infant mortality rate nationwide in the early 1930s was 6.8 percent, the rate for CMC births was 1.76 percent. The Center was also "a school of practical social science for the doctors, students and nurses who live there."[29] Tucker believed that the exposure to the "lives 'of the other half'" provided an unforgettable experience for students, who would

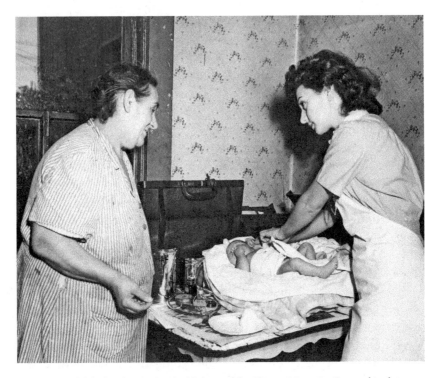

Figure 1.1 Published in the 1946 Annual Report of the Chicago Maternity Center, this photo was captioned: "Nursing service plays a vital role in the Center's aims not only to deliver a healthy baby, but to insure proper care after birth. Grandmother being taught how to care for newborn grandson, will pass on her knowledge to mother when she is up and about again." Photograph courtesy of the Chicago Maternity Center Collection, Northwestern Memorial Hospital Archives. Reprinted by permission.

no longer view the laboring mother as a "case," but rather as a "human being suffering both pain and poverty."[30]

BIRTH IN TRANSITION

Most importantly, the CMC provided medical students with an ample supply of "obstetric teaching material" at a time when women were increasingly opting for a hospital birth. DeLee believed that both populations were key to the growth of modern obstetrics, but they were invariably at odds with each other. "Obstetric practice is in a state of transition," DeLee declared in 1936. "It is necessary therefore to teach doctors and nurses now to care for maternity cases at home until there are enough good hospitals to deliver all the women. This cannot be expected for 20 years or more," he predicted.[31] His time frame proved surprisingly accurate; when he made this claim, 37 percent of all U.S. births took place in hospitals; twenty years later, 95 percent did.[32]

The problem was that the increasing proportion of women choosing hospital births resulted in a dwindling number of "sufficient clinical material." DeLee noted in 1941 that until recently, "we had enough patients for the teaching of all our hundreds of students, but the trek of the women in Chicago to hospitals for confinement is reducing the number who stay at home."[33] It appears illogical for the man held by many as responsible for the medicalization of childbirth to raise concern about an increase in hospital deliveries.[34] Yet his position on home birth was that it was more of a temporary training opportunity than an optimal method of delivery, and also a practice that was race- and class-based.[35] Hospital-based obstetric residencies did not exist until the 1930s and took over a decade to fully implement.[36] By trying to limit hospital births to first-rate training hospitals, he cornered the market on both home and hospital births, replacing midwives at home and poorly trained general practitioners in the hospital. And by utilizing a home birth clientele that was primarily poor, immigrant, or African American, he helped perpetuate a double standard in obstetrical method that would carry on well after his death in 1942. Patients who could not afford or were excluded from hospital births might be willing, even grateful, obstetrical guinea pigs—particularly if their only hospital options were limited to Cook County Hospital. A far higher percentage of white women gave birth in the hospital than women of color. In 1950, for example, 92.8 percent of white women and 57.9 percent of nonwhite women had their babies in the hospital rather than at home.[37]

Part of DeLee's success stemmed from the arrangements he made with local hospitals and several Midwestern universities to provide "all the formal training needed by a doctor to take examinations for the American Board of Obstetrics and Gynecology."[38] Hundreds of medical students from the University of Wisconsin, Northwestern University, and Chicago Medical School annually completed a three-week stay at the Maternity Center, while interns and residents stayed for six months to two years.[39] One of the first such residents recalled the Maternity Center was "flourishing" in 1949, a year in which nearly 4,000 home births took place under its direction, one out of every twenty deliveries in Chicago. "It was a lot of work," he remembers. "But people seemed to be active and happy."[40]

Tucker took every advantage to promote the success of the CMC training. "They enter these doors as students and become obstetricians," she declared in the 1952 annual report, illustrated with a photograph of the Chicago Maternity Center entrance. "Medical men and women famed in obstetrics have passed through these doors. And undoubtedly, some of those going out today will leave their mark on the future," she predicted.[41]

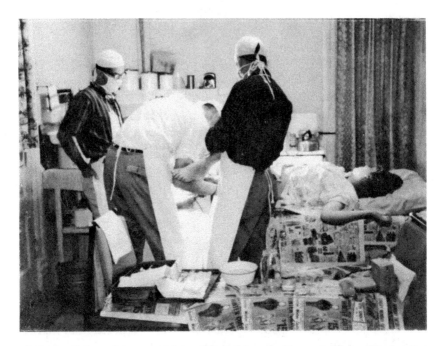

Figure 1.2 Photograph courtesy of the Chicago Maternity Center Collection, Northwestern Memorial Hospital Archives. Reprinted by permission.

How they made their mark on the future varied greatly. Brooks Ranney performed hundreds of home deliveries through the CMC as part of his residency program at Wesley Memorial Hospital beginning in 1945. He later served as the president of the American College of Obstetricians and Gynecologists (ACOG) from 1981 to 1983, where he spoke out against home birth. "Well do I know . . . the great inherent dangers associated with obstetric delivery at home," he declared in his inaugural presidential address. "Based upon that experience . . . I have chosen not to deliver a baby outside the environment of a thoroughly equipped and staffed hospital. Considering the overall welfare of the mother and baby, I could not choose otherwise."[42] Francis Brown worked at the CMC in the 1930s while studying at Rush Medical College. He would later open a home birth practice in New Hampshire, and according to midwife Carol Leonard, he was the only doctor in the state who was still doing home births in the 1970s. When Leonard inquired whether she might accompany him to births as a midwife in training, he thought it was a "great idea," and the apprenticeship launched her career.[43] Finally, Mayer Eisenstein worked at the CMC during its last days, inheriting some of the Center's pregnant clients when he opened his own home birth practice in Chicago. He would later train Kay Furey.

HOME AS HOSPITAL

Key to the success of the CMC program was its reconstruction of home birth as modern and hygienic. Annual reports, obstetric manuals, and media stories about the CMC revealed a setting more medical than domestic. Nurses were instructed to "secure conditions which closely resemble those of the maternity."[44] In effect, they were responsible for transforming the home into a hospital. Ideally, this process began two weeks before labor, when the nurse "tactfully" instructed families to clear the delivery room "of all unnecessary furniture, dust-catching bric-a-brac, hangings, rugs, and so on."[45] The 1944 edition of DeLee's *Obstetrics for Nurses* textbook, unlike previous editions, warned that "in some families the nurse may meet objections to what they term unnecessary preparations. The patient's mother was perhaps not delivered with much fuss and ado." What should a nurse do? "Here a little tact and explanation will clear the way. One cannot force advancement on people—one must smooth them into it."[46] Implicit in this instruction was the assumption that a modern home birth was in essence a medical one, characterized by the latest hygienic practices. And yet it was not always welcomed. "One may err with too much zeal," the textbook authors warned, "therefore the nurse should not make too great display of preparation, which might alarm the patient."[47]

With the onset of labor, the Maternity Center nurse sprang into action. "The nurse, like a general on the field of battle, frequently surveys the room to see if everything is in readiness," wrote DeLee, utilizing a militaristic analogy common in modern American nursing texts.[48] She helped to prepare the "patient" by shaving the pubic area and administering an enema. Births usually took place on the kitchen table rather than in the bedroom. All attendants and family members wore white masks, caps, gowns, and gloves. A photo essay in the 1948 annual report highlighted the obstetrical team attending to a birth in a "poor and cluttered home." Yet the camera lens is focused on the attendants gathered around the table. One assistant holds a floodlight in position so that the student can see as he guides the baby out of the birth canal. All clutter has been removed, and sterile medical supplies are visible in the foreground. Other reports referred to the attendants as "baby commandos" and to the Maternity Center as a " 'traveling hospital', whose specially trained teams bring tested delivery techniques into the home."[49] Thus, as hospital births were becoming the norm, home births began to resemble maternity wards.

Ironically, as this shift occurred, many women were starting to express dissatisfaction with the modern-day hospital maternity ward. As

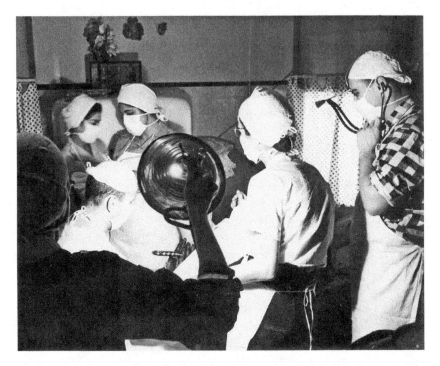

Figure 1.3 A birth scene published in *Today's Health Magazine*, April 1958. Note the doctor at the right wearing the DeLee-Hillis stethoscope. Photograph courtesy of the Chicago Maternity Center Collection, Northwestern Memorial Hospital Archives.

the percentage of hospital births increased, so too did complaints about unpleasant, mechanical, even traumatic experiences. In 1958, the *Ladies' Home Journal* published a disturbing article entitled "Cruelty in Maternity Wards." Growing numbers of middle-class women sought to avoid practices such as being involuntarily drugged and strapped down while in labor.[50]

In Chicago, a handful of local medical professionals representing general practitioners, pediatricians, and obstetricians responded to women's complaints by repackaging home birth as safer, more natural, and the antithesis of hospital birth. Some of these doctors had received their obstetrical training through the CMC. But in their own practices they focused on home birth's long-term advantages to mother and child rather than on its benefits to the medical community. Herbert Ratner, Robert Mendelsohn, and Gregory White all supported the idea that the best place for women to give birth was at home. In addition to their similar training and beliefs, they all served on the original Medical Advisory Board of the La Leche League.

BUILDING BETTER MOTHERS: MARIAN TOMPSON
AND THE LLL

By the mid-1950s, DeLee's vision of hospital birth had been achieved; 95 percent of women were giving birth in the hospital, compared to about 50 percent in 1940. At the same time, the rate of breastfeeding had dramatically decreased from 38 percent in 1948 to a mere 18 percent in 1956.[51] Even the CMC did not advocate breastfeeding.[52] But thanks to a group of mothers living in a Chicago suburb, that minority found its voice through the creation of La Leche League. The idea for the organization originated when Marian Tompson and Mary White sat under a tree breastfeeding their babies at a picnic in a Chicago suburb in the summer of 1956. They had become fast friends after Mary White's husband Gregory White delivered Tompson's fourth child at home the previous year. Together, they brainstormed about how to make breastfeeding more manageable for all women. Within months they had formed LLL, along with five friends. All were white, middle-class Roman Catholics active in the Christian Family Movement (a social justice organization) and interested in natural childbirth and breastfeeding. These seven women would give birth to and raise fifty-three children.[53]

Though LLL would later caution against "mixing causes," these founders saw a direct connection between birth experience and breastfeeding.[54] Both birth and infant feeding had been taken over by scientific "experts" in the twentieth century, which they felt had been detrimental to the mother–infant bond.[55] Even the name "La Leche League" hinted at the connection between birth and breastfeeding. The founders were having trouble coming up with an appropriate name, believing that anything with the word *breast* in it would be too controversial and difficult, if not impossible, to advertise. Dr. White often gave his home birth clients medals from a shrine honoring a Spanish madonna, "Nuestra Señora de la Leche y Buen Parto," which meant "Our Lady of Happy Delivery and Plentiful Milk."[56] Women who experienced a "happy delivery" (by which they meant medication free) were more likely to successfully breastfeed, because they would be awake and aware after the baby was born.

Women were also more likely to successfully breastfeed if they gave birth outside of the hospital. Chicago pediatrician and self-proclaimed "medical heretic" Robert Mendelsohn claimed that "unless a new mother puts up a hell of a fight . . . her baby is immediately swept away to that concentration camp known as the newborn nursery."[57] Many women complained of being physically separated from their newborn for hours after the birth, and being told that bottle feeding was better for their baby than breastfeeding. As a long-term member of the LLL Medical Advisory Board, Mendelsohn's pediatric expertise lent credibility to the claim that hospital births could have a negative impact on an infant's health. "For the vast majority of families, there is far less risk in a home birth than in a hospital birth," he argued.[58]

LLL founder Marian Tompson agreed with Dr. Mendelsohn. "Without a doubt, having a baby at home is at least as safe as a hospital birth, and in most situations, home birth is safer."[59] While she had no scientific degree to back up her opinion, her expertise came both from her knowledge of CMC statistics and from her own experience birthing the last four of her seven children at home. "It never occurred to me when expecting my first baby that I would ever want to have a baby at home. All I wanted then was natural childbirth."[60] But her negative hospital experiences convinced her that natural childbirth was really only possible at home.

While many associate the concept of "natural childbirth" with the method formulated by Fernand Lamaze—and by the 1970s the increasingly popular "Lamaze" classes were virtually synonymous with natural childbirth—Tompson's generation was more influenced by the work of British obstetrician Grantly Dick-Read. He introduced his childbirth method in 1933 with the publication of his first book, *Natural Childbirth*. In that and his 1944 *Childbirth Without Fear*, he posited that pain in childbirth was not physiological, but was instead rooted in fear. The solution was not anesthesia but preparation and education. Over 95 percent of women, he argued, are capable of experiencing childbirth without unbearable pain. He contended that his techniques enabled women to feel a "deep sense of satisfaction and joy in bearing children" rather than dread. "It is the right of every woman to be given that opportunity of learning how to make childbirth a happy event and not a hardship."[61]

Tompson remembers reading an article about Grantly Dick-Read in the *Ladies' Home Journal* when she was fifteen years old. "I have to lay it all at the foot of Grantly Dick-Read," she explained of her involvement in the breastfeeding and home birth movements. Though she was too young to fully absorb the impact of Dick-Read's message at the time, she realized later that this early exposure had paved the way for her later activism.[62]

When Tompson learned that Dick-Read would be stopping in Chicago in 1957 to talk to physicians and promote his work, she asked if he would be willing to come to the suburb of Franklin Park to speak to the newly formed La Leche League. "As women who had unmedicated births because of his book, we were very eager to meet him," she explained.[63] She was initially disappointed by his response, in which he suggested a public rather than a private talk, and a speaking fee of $700. Where would she find that amount of money, or a large enough audience? The group printed up fliers and sent them to anyone they thought might be interested. "To our amazement, we ended up filling the 1250-seat Franklin Park High School auditorium with people who came from three states" and raised far more money than the speaker fee. Attendants not only listened to the elderly British doctor but also watched, many in disbelief, a graphic film of three unmedicated births.[64] The high turnout suggested that many women were dissatisfied with the current state of childbirth.

Along with the $700 check, Tompson sent Dick-Read her profound gratitude for his visit. "Judging from the many excited and congratulatory phone calls I've been receiving today, your visit last evening to Franklin Park will long be remembered," she wrote. "To us it was an inspiring evening because we realized how great is the demand of our young men and women for a philosophy of childbirth and motherhood," Dick-Read responded enthusiastically. "My wife joins me in sending our gratitude."[65] In addition, the extra funds enabled the League to print information sheets about breastfeeding to mail to the steady stream of letter writers seeking advice. These sheets, in turn, led to the first version of their manual, *The Womanly Art of Breastfeeding*, printed in a series of loose-leaf folders and sold as a "course by mail."[66] The manual was turned into a book that has sold over two million copies.[67]

Tompson's exposure to the ideas of Grantly Dick-Read clashed with the realities of giving birth in the United States in the 1950s. Dick-Read assured his readers that childbirth was "an ecstasy of accomplishment that only women who have had babies naturally appreciate."[68] Children's author Cathleen Schurr affirmed these ideas in her 1953 book describing natural birth as "the supreme moment in a woman's life."[69] But as sociologist Barbara Katz Rothman noted in her ground-breaking study, *In Labor: Women and Power in the Birthplace*, Dick-Read's approach "failed in the United States because it did not prepare women for the social situation they had to face in labor."[70] Taken out of the British context, the Read method sometimes increased tension for the laboring woman. "While Dick-Read's book and method appealed to many American women," Rothman wrote, "the Americanization of Dick-Read was, in practice, something of a disaster."[71]

Tompson's hospital birth experiences support this claim. Her obstetrician had never heard of Grantly Dick-Read and had never observed an unmedicated birth, though he allowed her to give it a try for her first birth in 1950. It was a 36-hour labor "and the doctor was a little unhappy because, as he reminded me, if I was knocked out he could just slip in those forceps and have that baby out in a minute." The actions of the hospital staff, which included throwing a sheet over her head ("since women were knocked out for delivery, [nurses] were used to just concentrating on the other end"), strapping her wrists to the delivery table, and whisking her baby off to the nursery as soon as she was born prevented her from enjoying the experience. Her close proximity to the delivery room while she was in labor, fully cognizant for so many hours, enabled her to overhear what doctors and nurses were saying to drugged women.[72] "It frightened me to death because these women were all . . . yelling, screaming, and I heard one attendant say 'if you don't keep quiet I'm going to walk out of here and leave you alone.' Well I had never heard one adult talk to another like that. It was just frightening to me."[73] Tompson began to understand the impact of setting on the birthing experience. As she later explained, "the only thing I didn't like about having a baby was where I had to have it."[74] That changed after she discovered Dr. Gregory White.

THE LLL MEDICAL ADVISORY BOARD DOCTORS

White had studied under Dr. Herbert Ratner in the Department of Family and Community Medicine at Loyola University, and later opened up a family practice in Franklin Park. Like the Tompsons, Gregory and Mary White had their first three babies in the hospital and then opted for a home birth for the fourth, attended by Ratner in 1950. The birth went well, inspiring the two doctors to advocate a return to physician-assisted home births.[75] The Whites had seven more children at home with Gregory White as the medical attendant. Through word of mouth, his home birth practice evolved. "Some of my wife's friends who were patients of mine started asking me if I would deliver them at home too," White recalled. "I agreed. The thing slowly built through the years."[76] By 1977, approximately 80–90 percent of his deliveries took place in homes.[77] Over the course of his career he would attend over 5,000 births.[78]

White became a popular home birth doctor in part because of his bedside manner. "He sat with me through my whole labor," Kay Furey recalled. "I called him at two in the morning and I didn't deliver until late that evening." And yet, he stayed out of the way. "He almost never came into my bedroom. He would sit in the living room, read the paper, do his business, whatever, and my husband and I would labor in the bedroom."[79] He did this intentionally, explaining that the best birth attendant is one "who is willing to sort of fade into the wallpaper and let the couple do their thing, as long as everything is going well."[80] Marian Tompson remembers that "coming across Dr. Gregory White . . . was a gift beyond measure!" When he delivered her fourth baby in 1955, he charged $100 for a hospital delivery and $125 for a home birth, the difference most likely due to the extra time commitment involved.[81] Mayer Eisenstein, who apprenticed with White, noted that "he was the most patient person in the world and could make everyone feel comfortable. The simplicity of his techniques amazed me. He would watch and watch and watch at a birth, just really watch what was happening."[82]

White's appeal went beyond simply patience. Along with his mentor, Dr. Ratner, he believed passionately that the process of childbirth (and breastfeeding) cemented the mother–child relationship and strengthened family ties, thereby creating better mothers. "I think that those of you who have felt it and watched it know that the joy of childbirth gets motherhood off to a running start," he said at the first LLL convention in 1964. "Certainly there are many good mothers, many happy women who are not mothers who have never experienced the joy of childbirth, but those who have are unanimous in their testimony that this does help them to get to a quicker, easier, better start towards being a good mother."[83] His audience of breastfeeding advocates surely agreed.

Then White took it a step further. Childbirth, ideally a natural childbirth, restored maternal feelings to those who appeared to have lost them. "There are many, many little girls growing up in homes where [maternal feelings and practices] are hard to learn." It was 1964, a year after the publication of Betty Friedan's *Feminine Mystique* and a time when an increasing number of women were challenging traditional gender roles. White was among those who saw this as detrimental to the American family. "They are finding it hard to learn to be a mother perhaps because their own mother isn't home." White observed that many girls would come to marriage "with no particular conscious desire to ever be a mother." The solution? "These girls need the experience of birth desperately. For some of you this was just the last block in the building of motherhood which prepared you to take the baby in your arms and nurse it. But for some girls this experience of childbirth has to be nearly the whole building of motherhood in them."[84] It was thus crucial that they be active participants in their own labor.

Dr. Ratner spoke on mothering at the 1964 LLL convention. He argued that motherhood offered "an opportunity for growth." Taking an explicitly pronatalist slant, he declared that "three children nurture motherhood more than one. Each mothering experience enriches."[85] The problem was that the anxiety-producing hospital experience threatened to discourage women from having more children. 1964 marked the last year of the baby boom; the increasing liberalization of abortion, women's embrace of the birth control pill, and negative publicity for hospital births struck Ratner and White as indicative of unwelcome change to the family structure. As practicing Catholics, they felt that something had to be done to strengthen the foundation of family and motherhood. As doctors, what they felt comfortable critiquing was physicians' "growing indifference to person and

life."[86] An increasing emphasis on technology and intervention had super-
seded the true meaning of human reproduction, which they sought to
restore.

All three doctors on the LLL Medical Advisory Board, Ratner, White,
and Mendelsohn, believed that home birth would strengthen the relationship between mother and child as well as encourage certain women
to have more children. And Tompson, as president and spokeswoman for
LLL, was an effective promoter of this pronatalist message. "I really enjoy
being a mother," she declared in her 1975 keynote address at the Iowa
LLL area meeting. She could not identify with the messages promoted
in "*The Feminine Mystique*, followed later by other books in which women
were feeling they had been cheated biologically because they had to be the
bearers of children and they had to mother these children."[87] She initially
felt "out of step," perhaps just sort of a "dumb, warm animal-type who really
doesn't know any better, who isn't in tune with what's really important in
the world." But the more she thought about it, the more she believed that
she was simply experiencing "a different kind of motherhood, a different
concept of motherhood, and a different experience of motherhood."[88] She
was the perfect embodiment of the formula for motherhood promoted by
Drs. White, Ratner, and Mendelsohn. They, in turn, provided the authority
and expertise to convince LLL members that what they were doing was
medically safe.

The League's very success ironically proved instrumental in sidelining
home birth within the organization. As the LLL expanded beyond Franklin
Park, the demographics of its membership changed, and not all members
had access to or even an interest in home birth. "We were not very helpful
because we had no idea what the situations were in different localities,"
Tompson explained. One chapter of *The Womanly Art of Breastfeeding* focused on childbirth but made no mention of alternatives to hospital birth
(though it did warn that "at the hospital you may need to be prepared to assert yourself, in a nice way" in order to breastfeed).[89] When asked at the biennial convention in 1966 whether La Leche League preferred "that home
deliveries not be brought up at meetings," Tompson claimed it wasn't a political issue. "The only reason we don't usually mention it at meetings is
that most mothers can't have a home delivery in their locale, so, you know,
what's the sense of even talking about it? . . . We felt that it does no good to
have women interested in this possibility if they can't get it anyway."[90] By
that year, there were 430 LLL groups in existence; within ten years, this
would grow to 3,000.[91]

Tompson's statement attested to the fact that Chicago in the 1960s
remained unique in offering women the option of home birth. Well before
home birth gained popularity as a countercultural practice in the United

States, Chicago provided an alternative to residents who wished to stay out of the hospital. The CMC was still in operation. The LLL, while becoming increasingly reticent to directly advocate home birth, relied on the visibility and authority of White, Mendelsohn, and Ratner to promote out-of-hospital birth as a strategy for successful breastfeeding. Both organizations provided a scientific rationale for staying out of the hospital during this time.

THE DEMISE OF THE CMC

This decade would see the practice of obstetrics become firmly entrenched in the hospital. In the 1960s, the number of CMC births dropped precipitously. After peaking at close to 4,000 births in 1949, the number hovered at around 3,000 between 1957 and 1962.[92] By the time the Center closed in 1973, numbers were down to about 1,000 per year. Two factors help to explain the decline. The passage of Medicaid in 1965 enabled more poor women to deliver in a hospital, which for most Americans had become the standard and culturally desired place to give birth. And racism, poverty, and urban decline dramatically altered the Near West Side neighborhood where the Maternity Center was located, as well as the surrounding neighborhoods. In 1930 the population there was 78 percent white; in 1960 it was 0.5 percent white.[93] The neighborhood remained poor, but massive black migration during the postwar period and the resulting "white flight" from urban areas heightened segregation and exacerbated race relations.[94] Deteriorating conditions, poverty, and crime took a major toll on the community and on the CMC.

Dr. Tucker started having difficulty recruiting and keeping medical students (primarily white and middle class), who appeared increasingly uncomfortable working in the neighborhood. "Please, in no way, embarrass students who have left the Center between February 21 to March 6," she wrote to the Associate Dean of Northwestern University Medical School in 1971. "Dr. Miller was frightened by a brick thrown by a policeman, and left because he was afraid to stay. Dr. Buckley found the Center intolerable, and left."[95] In a later interview, Tucker explained that the decline of the Maternity Center was due in part to the fact that "medical students were afraid to go out in the homes."[96] Fear was exacerbated by sensationalized media coverage of Maternity Center births. "Rain beat hard against the window, and thunder echoed thru the room, heralding the infant's birth in the South Side slum apartment he would call home," began an article about a Maternity Center birth in the *Chicago Tribune* in 1971. "Roaches crawled along the wall molding far above him, and below, the floor was dotted with black gummy spots."[97] While DeLee had touted the benefits of teaching "good routine obstetrics" in the "poorest hovel" back in 1931, the racism and violence of the 1960s had turned any romantic notions of home birth into "moral" panic.

Students who went through the CMC training in the mid-1960s affirm these media depictions. Tim Hunter remembers the Center in 1968 as a "dump of a building."[98] David Kerns, who trained alongside Hunter, described their residence (Booth House, around the corner from the CMC) as "about as cozy as a meat locker." The CMC clinic, where patients went for prenatal checkups, "exuded all the ambience and charm of a bus station," he noted. It was also typically jam-packed. Pregnant women were "crammed side by side" on benches or "upright against the walls."[99]

While the CMC and dormitory buildings were in bad shape, they were nothing compared to the conditions of some of the patients' homes. Bob B., who was there in 1965, writes that his most memorable experience was "visiting the eighth floor of a southside high rise. Wearing our whites, we raised our black bags over our heads to announce who we were. The elevator, as usual for the building we understood, was not working. Apartment walls punched with holes, doors all on broken hinges. Taking a break on the entry porch, we could hardly hear each other because of the din from the overcrowded basketball court below."[100] Michele W. was a resident from Wesley Memorial Hospital who worked at the Center in the mid-1960s. "On several occasions while visiting patients 'on the district' we had our cars vandalized, dealt with the irate parents of teenage parturients, and of course had to contend with the ferocious Chicago weather."[101]

These students witnessed the city becoming swept up in the civil rights movement. In the summer of 1966, Martin Luther King established the headquarters for the Southern Christian Leadership Conference in a tenement building a few miles west of the CMC.[102] From there, he led a campaign to end racial segregation and to draw attention to the poor living conditions in Chicago's black neighborhoods. Though his campaign primarily focused on housing discrimination, King also drew attention to racial inequalities in health care, in particular the high infant mortality rate in black low-income neighborhoods. "Of all forms of discrimination and inequalities, injustice in health is the most shocking and inhuman," he said. "It is more degrading than slums, because slums are a psychological death while inequality in health is a physical death."[103]

When King initiated a series of marches throughout the city for open housing, riots erupted on Chicago's west side and interrupted its home delivery service. "We were in the area that was in trouble," Tucker explained. "It took courage on the part of the doctors and nurses to work during this particular time."[104] The city appeared to "teeter on the edge of disaster."[105] Marchers, including King, were struck by bottles and rocks.

The real death knell for the Chicago Maternity Center, however, was not rioting but urban renewal. The construction of the Dan Ryan Expressway in 1957 divided Maxwell Street and effectively tore the community apart. Like many urban freeway projects enabled by the 1956 Interstate Highway Act, the Dan Ryan benefited primarily white suburban commuters at the expense of primarily black urban neighborhoods. "For too long the history of urban renewal and highway clearance has been marked by the repeated removal of black citizens," noted members of Baltimore's Relocation Action Movement in 1968.[106] The Dan Ryan Expressway was clearly one of those projects.[107] Then, in the mid-1960s, Tucker learned that the CMC building was slated for demolition when Mayor Daley chose the historic Near West Side neighborhood as the location for a new campus for the University of Illinois.[108] Hull House was also in the path of destruction, but was partially saved by virtue of its status as a National Historic Landmark.

PRENTICE WOMEN'S HOSPITAL

Good news tentatively lay ahead for the future of the Center, however. Chicago Wesley Memorial Hospital, Passavant Memorial Hospital, and Northwestern University Medical School had recently partnered to develop a new women's hospital on the campus of Northwestern University Medical Center. Arthur Halland, the president of the CMC board, announced in 1967 that "considerable progress" had been made toward the construction of the new building, to be called Prentice Women's Hospital, which would include space for the Chicago Maternity Center and "facilities for the continuance of our home delivery service."[109]

As plans developed, Tucker sensed that the absorption of the CMC into this new facility would weaken the historic Center. David Danforth, chair of Ob/Gyn at Northwestern, predicted in 1970 that Prentice "will be the newest and, excepting the Cook County Hospital, the largest obstetric-gynecologic facility in Chicago." The "high patient volume" would attract scientists and specialists in obstetrics, as well as allow for "a significant increase in the size of the medical school class" at Northwestern. While in the past, Northwestern's medical students had been assigned to multiple hospitals as well as to the CMC, "the new hospital will absorb the senior program entirely, and will also be capable of providing clinical teaching, comfortably, for 20 students."[110]

Tucker was right to be concerned. Immediately before a new resident was slated to begin a rotation at the CMC, she received bad news.

"I was knocked off my base by the sudden withdrawal of Wesley residents," Tucker wrote to Melvyn Bayly, Chief of Obstetrics at the hospital in late June of 1972. "I wish to assure you that I am committed to the cause of home obstetrics, and fully aware of the adverse position of organized medicine, and many social agencies."[111] She wrote an additional plea to Danforth at Northwestern, whom she blamed for the decision to end the affiliation with the Maternity Center. "It seems absolutely necessary that I again draw your attention to the fact that the CMC cannot operate without one full time resident who lives at the CMC."[112] At almost seventy-five years old, Tucker was also concerned about what would happen upon her retirement.

Despite attempts by consumer groups and home birth advocates to save the CMC, Northwestern University closed it in December of 1973, claiming it was no longer cost effective. Many more laboring patients could be attended to in the new hospital than if medical workers were dispersed all over the city. In the hospital setting, medications could be used to speed up labor, shortening the length of time a patient would need to be in a delivery room. In the home, labor was subject only to nature.

The construction of Prentice Women's Hospital marked more than the end of the Maternity Center. Its design, according to preservation campaigners that attempted to save the building, "changed the course of modern hospital design" and "helped redefine patient- and family-centered care."[113] The brutalist style building, a clover-shaped tower, featured a predominance of exposed concrete intended to communicate strength and functionality. Patients were gathered in four small groups on each floor in curved sections that resembled the clover leaves. At each floor's center lay a nursing station, where staff could easily observe all four sections. "They were called pods," explained a postpartum nurse who worked there in 1981. "There were 12 beds in a pod. You take a piece of pie and you cut it into four quarters and that's what you've got. In the middle of the pie was the nursing station. At night all the babies, even the breastfeeding babies were taken into the nursery where they were weighed and washed and everything."[114]

The new design brought mothers and even fathers closer to their babies, suggesting that hospital birth could be family-centered. But closer proximity under the gaze of hospital staff, situated at the center of all activity, did not actually replicate the home birth model. If anything, it more closely resembled the panopticon structure designed by Jeremy Bentham in the late eighteenth century, in which a watchman at the center of a building is able to observe all inmates located around the perimeter. Rather than enabling privacy between a mother, father, and child, it imposed a higher level of surveillance and intervention.

HOMEFIRST

The real legacy of the CMC was not Prentice Hospital, but the continued practice of home birth that flourished in the city's suburbs. Many of the medical students and interns who had trained at the CMC later became advocates and practitioners of home births nationwide. Mayer Eisenstein, for example, provided a crucial link between the CMC and the growing home birth community in the 1970s and 80s. He studied pediatrics with LLL advisory board member Mendelsohn, as well as obstetrics with Gregory White and Beatrice Tucker during her last year at the CMC. "I would go to her house every Tuesday night and discuss obstetrics with her," he remembered. "She was history and I was witnessing her last doctoring days. I just couldn't let go."[115] When the CMC closed, Eisenstein inherited many of its clientele, particularly those who could afford to pay.

In 1973, Kay Furey, then working as a LLL leader, received a phone call from Eisenstein. He was about to open his own practice (which he called "Homefirst") and wanted to hire a LLL leader to work in the office and counsel his patients on breastfeeding. "So I came to work as a receptionist. I didn't know anything medical at that point," she recalled. Within a year, she was accompanying Mayer to clients' homes to provide breastfeeding support, and shortly after that, she began assisting him at home births. "One thing led to another . . . then I started catching the babies."[116] Furey remembers this as an exciting time; Eisenstein was just learning about obstetrics, and "I learned along with him." She kept an obstetrical log, carefully recording each birth—including the mother's age and race, street address, health history, and outcome. In the early 1980s, she and Eisenstein attended approximately ten births per month. Mothers were overwhelmingly white and averaged 25–35 years in age.[117]

The Homefirst practice expanded quickly; by the time Furey left in 1989 to become a nurse-practitioner midwife, there were six doctors in the practice who had delivered approximately 5,000 babies at home.[118] While doing his residency in Milwaukee, Dr. Paul Schattauer met a local home birth doctor who recommended a medical rotation in Chicago with Eisenstein. "That sealed the deal," he said of his ten Chicago births.[119] "Finding Homefirst was like finding a gold mine! These doctors are happy people who enjoy their work. . . . I have found the family practice aspects of medicine that I was looking for and I get to experience those close family relationships that happen at birth."[120] Schattauer worked with Homefirst for twenty-three years and delivered over 1,000 babies at home. Dr. Mark Zumhagen first encountered Eisenstein when his wife was pregnant with their third son. "It never entered my mind that I would become involved in a practice such as Homefirst until I became involved with the practice as a parent," he reflected. His wife was more relaxed during her labor, and he was not made to feel like an intruder "as I had felt during our previous hospital births."[121] Other Homefirst associates included George Dietz, who was married to one of Dr. Ratner's daughters; Dr. Peter Rosi, who had trained midwives in Alaska for several years before Eisenstein recruited him to join Homefirst; and Dr. Jean Flood. Flood first learned of the organization from a fundraiser at her daughter's school, where someone was auctioning off a Homefirst home birth. She contacted Eisenstein to request an interview and was hired on the spot. "No one who works for Homefirst has lukewarm feelings about his or her job. . . . Dr. Eisenstein has set up a brilliant and exemplary practice. I am thrilled to be a part of it!"[122]

Part of Eisenstein's brilliance was his ability to successfully promote home birth as both safe and meaningful. "I think Mayer Eisenstein should be given credit for sustaining homebirth and sustaining doctors' interest in Tucker's vision," remarked his colleague Paul Schattauer. Eisenstein appeared several times on both the *Phil Donahue Show* and *The Oprah Winfrey Show*. He also hosted a weekly radio program, "Family Health Forum," on Saturday mornings, along with monthly film screenings. "The home birth that we're talking about in 1986 is not the same home birth as 50–100 years ago," Eisenstein remarked in a radio interview. "1986 home birth brings advanced technology to the home," he explained. Homefirst doctors brought oxygen, resuscitation equipment, and over 100 different medications in case of a medical emergency.[123] "High Tech! Home Touch!" he announced in a patient flier. "Now you can have all the advantages of both a traditional home environment and modern childbirth technology."[124]

Eisenstein made clear that he saw his practice as a continuation of the CMC and Dr. Tucker's home birth legacy. The combination of home comfort and modern technology was pioneered, he believed, by Tucker. He created a medical fellowship and annual awards in her name, explaining that "Dr. Tucker was very influential in the forming of Homefirst's philosophy." [125]

But many people noted a different style between CMC births and those of Eisenstein, suggesting two different models of home birth. "It was very medical," Kay Furey noted of her second birth at home with CMC personnel. "If you're having your first baby you're on a table."[126] Another woman, Kathy, had her first child with Dr. Tucker and the second with Eisenstein, noting that Tucker wanted the home births to be as much like the hospital setting as possible. "Two nurses came to my house wearing masks. We all had to wear caps covering our hair . . . . I was free to walk around, eat, and do whatever I felt like doing but when the time came to push I had to get up on the kitchen table." Kathy's second baby was born in 1976, and since the Maternity Center had closed, Tucker sent her to Dr. Eisenstein, who delivered her next three babies at home.[127] Tucker's daughter-in-law had both Tucker and a young Eisenstein at her birth. "Dr. Eisenstein was a new doctor and so laid back. Dr. Tucker was so much more the sterilizing hospital type. Of course both of them treated their patients very well, it was just different. I'd say that Dr. Tucker brought forward the best of the past and Dr. Eisenstein was able to pick up on that and expand it into his own style."[128]

Eisenstein, like DeLee before him, was quick to capitalize on the capability of physicians to make home birth a safe experience. But he had his eye on a different type of clientele than the typical CMC patient. The middle-class consumer—who could afford to pay for the service—created a new market for physicians interested in home birth. "I like how consumers are getting smarter!" remarked Dr. Schattauer. "Those consumers who have properly researched all the options are the ones who return as our patients," he added. They were interested not just in safety, but in comfort. The Homefirst delivery team, Eisenstein explained, usually a doctor and a nurse, "work towards making the mother as comfortable as possible."

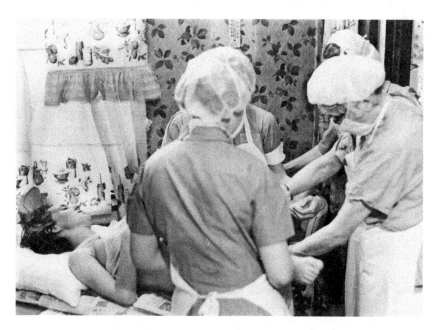

Figure 1.4 This photograph appeared in an article by Lois Baur, "The Woman the Babies Meet First," *Chicago's American*, March 1, 1966. It was captioned: "Lily, a delicately boned 22-year old mother-to-be, was moved from the rollaway bed to the kitchen table for a pelvic examination conducted by Dr. Tucker, medical director of the Chicago Maternity Center. Ten hours after this picture was taken Lily gave birth to a 7 lb. 7 oz. son, Daniel Clyde." Photograph courtesy of the Chicago Maternity Center Collection, Northwestern Memorial Hospital Archives.

They provided encouragement and input, but stressed that the mother controlled the scenario.[129]

At the very historical moment that hospital birth was becoming the norm in the United States, two different rationales for resisting that trend emerged in Chicago. In his quest to elevate the field of obstetrics, Joseph DeLee sought greater opportunities to train medical students. He believed that the optimal place for students to practice their skills was in the home. But in order to justify the practice and raise funds for his CMC, he needed to provide evidence that home birth was both safe and cost effective. As part of this promotion, he carefully instructed nurses, students, and doctors to transform the "poorest hovel" into a modern maternity ward. This version of home birth was far from oppositional to hospital birth; instead, it paved the way for greater acceptance of a medical model of birth.

As DeLee's promotion of medicalized birth became more accepted, it also triggered a backlash. The desire on the part of a group of white middle-class women to breastfeed resulted in a new justification for home birth, one that focused on celebrating motherhood. The most effective way to promote a strong bond between mother and child, they argued, was to stay out of the hospital.

Despite the distinction between these two rationales, there remained a philosophical and practical connection: the Chicago Maternity Center. The same program that created a future president of ACOG who spoke out against home birth, Brooks Ranney, also inspired organizations like Eisenstein's Homefirst. Eisenstein recognized the simmering discontent among many middle-class women about hospital practices. "We were never a practice of promotion, we were a practice of attraction," he told his coworkers.[130] Women like Marian Tompson and Kay Furey were looking for opportunities to avoid another unpleasant hospital experience, and doctors like Eisenstein and White provided it for them. Furey, in turn, would become a midwife, which rapidly became the most common type of attendant at a home birth beginning in the 1970s.

The fact that both types of home birth flourished for decades—and shared practitioners and some clients—underscores the importance of challenging the oppositional model of home versus hospital. The CMC originated in the dreams of an obstetrician whose long-term goal was to make hospital birth ubiquitous. And DeLee came close to achieving that. But he also provided experience and evidence to those who began with the premise that home birth could be safe, effective, and scientific—and turned it into a meaningful, revolutionary experience for families, rather than merely a teaching tool for the practitioner.

From inner-city tenements to Franklin Park colonials, women's actual birth experiences in Chicago probably varied as much as the setting itself.

But the promotion of home birth by individual obstetricians, pediatricians, breastfeeding activists, and midwives ensured that the practice would continue well after the destruction of the CMC. Decades before home birth became associated with either feminism or the counterculture, it was well ensconced in the city and suburbs of Chicago.

CHAPTER 2

⤫

Middle-Class Midwifery

Transforming Birth Practices in Suburban Washington, D.C.

We did it because it was the right time, you know—there were so many people who were ducking out of the hospital because it had become so restrictive and so backward and they wanted something else.

—Marion McCartney, CNM, December 13, 2011

Thanks to the CMC and the LLL, home birth remained an established practice in Chicago well after it had disappeared in most cities. But by the 1970s, the home birth trend had taken root in other cities including Washington, D.C. Between 1970 and 1977, the number of out-of-hospital births there more than doubled, from 0.6 percent to 1.5 percent.[1]

Helen and John Morarre were one of the couples that contributed to the increase by choosing to stay at home for their daughter Robin's birth in April of 1975. As the soundtrack to *Godspell* played in the background, Helen labored in the second-floor bedroom in Jessup, Maryland, surrounded by six pots of daffodils. John, a junior high school band teacher, read passages from the Bible as a doctor and nurse monitored contractions.[2] "It was the most wonderful experience," exclaimed Helen. "There was no rush from home to hospital and no adjustment from hospital to home. Your baby and your husband are with you all the time. It's wonderful."[3] The Morarres chose to stay out of the hospital because they were Christian Scientists. Others, according to local midwife Fran Ventre, were "counter-culture people—some in communes, some single women. But a lot of them are very respectable middle-class people like myself," she added.[4]

This increase in home births paralleled a rise in consumer advocacy groups. LLL inspired the formation of one such group, the Home Oriented Maternity Experience in Washington, to provide support and information on home birth. H.O.M.E. and other, similar birth organizations of the 1970s focused not just on the place of birth but on the practitioner as well. For centuries, midwives had guided women through their births, and these consumer advocates believed it was time they made a comeback. Whether the midwife needed to be licensed and certified was up for debate and would become hotly contested.

Who were these Washingtonians who, seemingly overnight, developed an interest in home birth? And what circumstances led them to propose that midwives, rather than obstetricians, should be the primary birth attendants? "Everything was happening all at the same time," midwife Marion McCartney remembers. "Women were getting disgusted with being put to sleep and having a baby dragged out with forceps. So that was a good time for us. I mean it was the perfect time to become a midwife."[5]

Many of the D.C. area women attribute their "calling" to midwifery at least in part to their experiences as mothers and childbirth educators. They were the first generation able to take advantage of specialized education in the area, with the establishment of the nurse-midwifery program at Georgetown University in 1974. Their relationships with individual doctors, nurses, other midwives, and teachers also shaped their careers as well as the future path of midwifery. Together, they contributed to the nation's burgeoning home birth movement and helped to package it as a middle-class phenomenon.

NATURAL CHILDBIRTH IN WASHINGTON

On the cover of the Sunday, October 18, 1970 edition of the *Washington Post Potomac* magazine, newborn Erin Reilly posed with her parents, Mr. and Mrs. Paul J. Reilly, in the delivery room of Washington Hospital Center. Erin's father, a doctoral candidate in history at Georgetown University, dressed in hospital scrubs, has just untied his hospital mask and stares lovingly at his daughter. In this full cover photograph, he takes up most of the page, with wife and daughter offset to the bottom third, an indicator of the increasingly accepted—and central—role that fathers were starting to play at their children's births.[6] Across his chest was the title of this cover story: "A holy war rages over natural childbirth." Author Stephan Schwartz, who himself had just witnessed his own child being born at the same hospital, set out to determine why many D.C. area hospitals and obstetricians remained opposed to the idea of natural childbirth. Of the twenty-two area hospitals that had maternity wards in 1970, only eight allowed fathers in the delivery room, while eleven specifically banned them. "I do not like, and cannot understand this business of husbands wanting to be in the delivery room," declared Dr. Robert Nelson Jr., chairman of the D.C. Medical Society's obstetrics committee and former medical director of the Washington Planned Parenthood Association.[7] "There is less confusion, less chance of contamination, less traffic with fewer people (without him). This is, let me stress, an operating room."[8] He believed that the easiest method of delivery "is one in which the woman is heavily sedated."[9]

Nelson was not alone, the American Society for Psychoprophylaxis (ASPO, a.k.a. Lamaze), formed in 1960, noted. The organization considered the nation's capital to be a "heavy medication area."[10] Many local women, including my mother, gave birth while unconscious in the 1960s. Dr. Josiah Sachs, vice-chairman of the department of obstetrics and gynecology at Holy Cross hospital, recalled that in 1968, 90 percent of the deliveries at his hospital were done "with the mother completely asleep and the father pacing the waiting room floor."[11] Marion McCartney, who observed hospital births in nursing school, remembers that "they would give them so many drugs in labor I was surprised they wouldn't fall out of bed."[12] By 1970 several organizations had begun to offer childbirth classes to expectant couples looking for a different experience, among them a local area chapter of ASPO, Childbirth Education Association, Inc., and Parent and Child, Inc. Stephan Schwartz and his wife signed up for the most popular of the three, ASPO, which offered six classes once a week. They were one of five couples to learn how to manage labor without medication from registered nurse and certified ASPO instructor Julie Boruff. "Several of the other prospective parents are as hip as others are straight," Schwartz wrote. "There seems to be no constant other than an open mind and a disaffection with the traditional American obstetrical scenario."[13]

Through word of mouth, couples learned which doctors and which hospitals were more supportive of Lamaze. Pam Bescher, the founder of the D.C. chapter of ASPO, noted how crucial obstetrical support was. "The key to the thing lies with the doctor. If he is supportive, you'll get through."[14] Al and Cheryl Diehl heard Dr. Donald Meek, an "unabashed proponent of the method," lecture on natural childbirth and "became convinced" that it was for them. They were one of some 20,000 couples in the D.C. area (and 400,000 nationwide) who were opting for unmedicated childbirth by 1971.[15] After rupturing Cheryl's amniotic sac while she was in labor at Georgetown University Hospital, Meek remarked to a reporter covering the birth, "the whole thing requires a tremendous amount of trust between doctor and patient. You know, many doctors don't like this method because it threatens them." Meek preferred open communication with his patients, which meant they had to be conscious. "I talk to my patients. It's a cooperative thing. It's almost a spiritual thing."[16] At thirty-seven years old, he had already delivered 2,000 babies and still "got a kick" out of it.

Meek, Besher, and Boruff were part of a highly organized group of advocates and professionals pushing to reform birth practices in the D.C. area through childbirth education. This involved offering classes not just for prospective parents, but also for prospective instructors. "We come away from our ASPO childbirth preparation classes feeling prepared and anxious for that big day," noted Jane Murphy in the local ASPO newsletter. "Our teachers seem to instill enthusiasm and confidence in us. They have a wealth of knowledge. . . . How did they become such all-around good teachers?" she asked in her column on teacher training. Those interested in becoming certified ASPO instructors had to possess an MD or RN degree or hold a degree in the sciences. Training included a handful of required seminars, birth observations, an exam, and written birth reports from both the trainee and the birthing couple.[17]

Many of those who went through this rigorous training for ASPO instructors found themselves radicalized in the process. Future midwife Alice Bailes wrote to the D.C. ASPO group that she felt "profoundly changed in several ways" after taking the training course in 1972. "My approach to childbirth is even more enthusiastic now than when I first started the application process for the training program. I'm afraid that you guys have been instrumental in turning me into a fanatic. I understand the absolute necessity for training for mother and father and child. Childbirth is a much broader experience now than it was in my mind before."[18] Her future midwifery business partner, Marsha Jackson, decided to train as an ASPO instructor because she had attended a hospital childbirth education class during her own pregnancy and was less than impressed. "I knew that I could do a better job preparing families for childbirth." Through her training with ASPO, she learned about the emerging home birth movement in the area and eventually began delivering babies at home as a certified nurse-midwife.[19]

Like La Leche League members in Chicago, this group of educators and birth reformers provided the organization and networking that launched a far more radical home birth movement in the D.C. area than its founders intended. As the editors of the *Washington Post Potomac* noted in their 1970 article, "despite the careful trappings of doctors advisory boards and such, this is at its core a movement of women. Regardless of the cookies-and-tea atmosphere, these organizations [ASPO and LLL] have power."[20] Part of their influence stemmed from the shared interest of many women in making childbirth and motherhood a positive, empowering experience. Many advocates believed that these organizations could join together to make that happen.

BEFORE THEY WERE MIDWIVES

Special Delivery, the newsletter of the professional and physicians divisions of Washington D.C. ASPO, suggests the extent to which ideas about natural childbirth, midwifery, and breastfeeding overlapped in the 1970s. "INFORMATION PLEASE," wrote Fran Ventre in the November 1972 issue. "For our next edition of *Special Delivery* I would like to include something about the International Confederation of Midwives." Aware that ASPO members had attended sessions and spoken with midwives, she asked them to send her their impressions. "I think that it would be of interest to all of us," she stated. In the same newsletter, she also reported on the La Leche League 1972 State Conference for the Blue Ridge-Potomac Area that had taken place the previous month. She and future lay midwife Tina Long were the only ASPO members to attend the conference. "I think it might be a good idea for all of us to keep in touch with what's happening in La Leche League and be aware of the recent medical information pertaining to breastfeeding, as our students frequently turn to us for their first questions on the nursing relationship."[21]

In addition to professional reasons to stay abreast of happenings in LLL, Ventre had personal ones; LLL had brought her much needed support when she struggled with breastfeeding her own children, and it was where she met her closest friend and professional partner, Esther Herman, who would become a local LLL leader. Together they created the aptly named childbirth advocacy group, H.O.M.E. (Home Oriented Maternity Experience), in the spring of 1974. Within seventeen months, H.O.M.E. had received more than 6,000 letters, mailed over 2,000 quarterly newsletters, and exceeded 1,000 members and thirty-five affiliated groups nationwide.[22] Newsletters reported on midwifery legislation, medical findings, conferences, and the history of childbirth. Volunteers answered the phone, responded to inquiries, and typed up copy from Herman's Takoma Park basement, as seen in Figure 2.1. Ventre hosted home birth preparation classes, similar in design to breastfeeding classes at LLL, in her Chevy Chase living room.

While pregnant in the summer of 1966, Ventre remembers meeting another pregnant woman at a swimming pool. "And she started telling me that she and her husband were going to these natural childbirth classes. And I'm sitting there and I'm thinking 'you've got to be crazy. You're going to go through that?' She said 'yeah, you want to come along with me?' And I said,

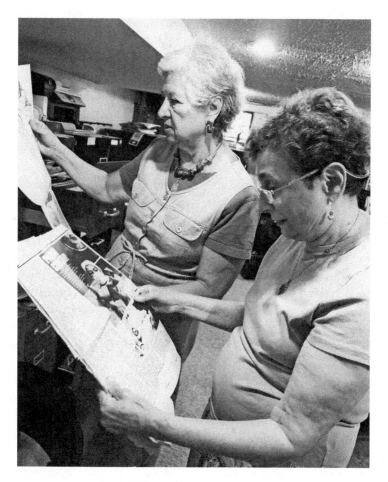

Figure 2.1 Fran Ventre and Esther Herman perusing old H.O.M.E. files in Herman's basement, July 22, 2011. Photograph by Wendy Kline. Reprinted by permission.

'I don't think so.' But I decided to go."[23] She ended up at Phyllis Stein's house in Wheaton, Maryland, an encounter that would change her life.

At twenty-one years old, Phyllis Stein had become the first-ever lay certified ASPO educator, in part because of a personal connection with ASPO founder Elizabeth Bing.[24] Stein had a different approach to childbirth than many ASPO teachers, in part because of her politics. "I was a hippie before there *were* hippies," she recalls. She was extremely bright; she entered Barnard College at the age of fifteen and graduated in three years. She married her college boyfriend and the two of them entered graduate school in physics at Rutgers. Stein quickly realized that while she was good at physics, she didn't find it personally rewarding. At the age of eighteen, she dropped out and got pregnant. She and her husband moved to Washington, D.C. for her husband's job, and she became involved in both La Leche League, after the birth of her first child in 1963, and ASPO. She learned about home birth from her friends in LLL and gave birth to her second son at home in 1966, shortly before Ventre showed up for her childbirth class.[25]

Ventre remembers that Stein showed a childbirth film that night in her class, a documentary circulated by Dr. Lamaze's chief assistant, Pierre Vellay. The twenty-four-minute film explained the psychoprophylactic method and then featured a live birth with Vellay in attendance.[26] "The woman was having a baby and she was smiling," Ventre recalled. "I said, 'Oh my God'. It was totally different than the film I had seen where they shave the woman and gave her an enema." After the class, she stayed after to talk to Stein, realizing that she had had a change of heart. She wanted to give birth naturally so that she could welcome her baby into the world. However, she was slated to deliver at Georgetown University Hospital, which did not allow fathers in the room. Stein told her that a student nurse could assist her with Lamaze breathing through the labor.[27] F.J. Ventre was born on February 2, 1966, two days after the "blizzard of '66" brought frigid temperatures and eighteen inches of snow to the "district of Siberia."[28] Ventre's husband was not allowed in the room, but she did have an unmedicated birth—and a painful delivery with forceps.

Ventre found herself with a young infant son and very little local support. Her parents had both passed away by the time she was a teenager. "I was in pain from sore nipples and exhausted since he nursed all the time and never slept."[29] Her pediatrician advised her to stop breastfeeding, assuming that she didn't have enough milk. In tears and determined to continue breastfeeding, she telephoned Phyllis Stein for advice. Stein suggested that she attend a La Leche League meeting that evening and arranged for someone to pick her up and take her there.[30] Sitting next to her at the meeting was Esther Herman, with her five-month-old daughter Rachel.

Herman was raised on a chicken farm in Petaluma, California, and studied child psychology at the University of California, Berkeley. In 1965 she moved to Takoma Park, one of the first Washington suburbs, with her husband and first child. The neighborhood, sometimes referred to as the "Berkeley of the East" or the "People's Republic of Takoma Park," attracted residents concerned with social issues and was the site of frequent protests.[31] Herman felt right at home. While pregnant with her second child, she ran into an old friend from Petaluma living nearby. "She told me about childbirth classes with this wonderful person named Phyllis Stein," Herman remembers. "I took a series of classes even though I was delivering in a military hospital. I thought it would be helpful. I had a really tough time with my first one so I thought this might make it easier."[32] Her first child was also delivered in a military hospital, where her husband was not allowed to be at the birth, and Herman was not allowed to hold her baby for twenty-four hours.[33] "It's because of her [Stein] that I ended up having my third child [and fourth] at home," Herman explains.[34] Stein's information and insights about birth enabled Herman to view what happened the second time more critically. "They let me hold my daughter for a few seconds," Herman says of Rachel Herman's birth in September of 1965, "but then they took her off to the nursery for 36 hours. By then she wasn't willing to nurse, and she lost weight until I got home."[35] Herman would never give birth in a hospital again.

Herman and Ventre became fast friends when they met at that La Leche League meeting in 1966. Both had taken childbirth classes with Phyllis Stein and felt empowered (and then frustrated) with their birth outcomes. Both struggled to nurse their infants, despite their desire to do so. "Esther was my lifeline," Ventre recalls.[36] Over the following decades, Herman would become very active in the LLL movement, training as a leader and holding regular meetings at her house. Ventre would become a midwife and would hold home birth meetings at her house. Along with other local women, they selected what they saw as the most advantageous aspects and opportunities of more conservative groups such as ASPO and LLL and pieced together their own version of childbirth reform. Ventre and Herman were rabble rousers, true to the spirit of Takoma Park.

At the time when Ventre and Herman met, the Washington area LLL was on the verge of exploding. In 1967, local membership had increased so dramatically that it needed a new state officer to handle new applications and new groups in the area.[37] By 1975, the area (designated "Blue Ridge/ Potomac") had seven districts, twenty-seven chapters, and eighty-eight local groups.

LLL state officers viewed the large number of chapters and groups in the D.C. area with guarded optimism. "We have watched Blue Ridge-Potomac LLL growing by leaps and bounds these past years with a feeling of pride, awe, and affection for the leaders and all the other mothers who have made it possible," they wrote in 1975. Such a dramatic increase, however, also required greater management. "As our family grows we find it necessary (sigh) to put our house in some semblance of order so that we will be working together more effectively," they continued. In order to facilitate greater communication and coherence, the state officers assembled a fifty-page manual that included a list of LLL policies on a "handy dandy reference sheet."[38]

According to LLL policy, leaders should follow guidelines when meeting with a new group member or when consulted by members of the local media. They needed to keep records of every group meeting, which were scheduled in a series of four classes for new members. And meetings were to be limited to women. Herman took issue with that policy, and the meetings at her home included fathers as well beginning in 1967 or 1968. "My group *was* the first one to welcome the dads."[39] Her husband referred to La Leche League as her "front organization," Herman recalls, "because one day there was a knock on the door and this couple was standing there. She was pregnant, he was with a scruffy beard, a long wool overcoat, a Russian newspaper under his arm, a Russian pin on his lapel, and he came in. And he said is this where the meeting is? *The* meeting. So they came in and he was the first man."[40] They had just moved back from the USSR, where the wife had been in the foreign service. "We have been close friends with this couple all of the years since. They attended every one of our family celebrations when they weren't out of the country for the foreign service," Herman recalls.[41]

Ventre similarly found herself limited by the constraints set upon her teaching methods by ASPO. ASPO founder Elizabeth Bing was supportive of natural childbirth, but only if it took place in the hospital. Originally, Ventre agreed. "I was confident that hospitals would eventually change and better consider the emotional needs of the childbearing family," she wrote. "But the hospitals did not change and continued to treat the natural processes of birth as a major surgical procedure. Change, I then decided, would not come from within the institutional establishment, but rather from outside channels of alternatives."[42] Her radicalized stance did not sit well with ASPO, which put her certification in jeopardy.[43]

This conflict was illustrated by her interactions with Dr. Meek, the local ASPO officer and the young obstetrician at Georgetown who loved delivering babies and was an avid supporter of natural childbirth. Ventre described him as "brash" and "handsome" but difficult. "He thought he was God's gift to women," she said. He lived around the corner from her home in Chevy Chase, and they often hosted ASPO film showings such as *The Story of Eric*. She remembers one evening when they walked home together, arguing in the street about home birth. He said to her, " 'you know, I don't like your homebirth stance.' He said, 'I don't think I'm going to send any of my patients to your childbirth classes.' I said, 'that's okay Dr. Meek, I won't refer any of my people in my childbirth classes to you, either.'"[44] This exchange (as recalled later by Ventre) underscores a dramatic shift in the power relations between consumers and obstetricians in the 1970s.[45] Ventre was well aware of her ability to attract a growing number of middle-class clientele interested in giving birth outside the hospital. Despite Meek's obstetrical expertise and his support of natural childbirth, he faced increasing competition from the alternative birth community.

A few years after this encounter, Ventre remembers another exchange with Meek. She got into an argument with him about home birth while attending a party at his house, and as she turned to leave, he called her back. " 'It's because of you people are having home birth,' he said. I said 'what do you mean because of me? It's not because of me. I just give information. And yeah if people wanted, that's their decision.' He said, 'because of you, my new wife wants me to deliver our child up there' [pointing to his up-stairs bedroom]. I said 'well good for her'. And he said something like, 'over my dead body'. So I said, 'have a nice day'. We parted. That was the last time I saw Donald Meek." Later, Ventre heard that Meek's wife had given birth not once, but twice, in their bedroom, supposedly accidentally.[46] Whether or not she remembers these stories entirely accurately, they suggest the increasing threat of the home birth movement to obstetrical authority. In the first exchange, Ventre reminds Meek of her power to send her nat-ural childbirth patients elsewhere. In the second exchange, it has become personal.

But not all obstetricians were opposed to home birth; in fact, a handful were instrumental in enabling it to happen safely. As in Chicago, Washington had its share of home birth doctors long after the majority of births took place in the hospital. Dr. James Brew and Dr. Ludwig DeVocht were two proponents and practitioners of home birth in the D.C. area. They trained many local women interested in learning midwifery skills, including Fran Ventre, Alice Bailes, Jan Epstein, and Marion McCartney, often after deliv-ering their babies. DeVocht delivered Alice Bailes' son at home in 1973. "And that was a lovely experience," she recalls.[47] She describes a "profound sense of delicious peace. . . . it was so satisfying, so different from the harsh hospital-imposed, twenty-four hours of separation from my daughter that I experienced immediately after she emerged."[48] Brew delivered Epstein's first child, Amy, in 1968 at Washington Hospital Center. Shortly thereafter, "I went to a home birth him and it was spectacular," she remembered. "I was struck by the simplicity of it. No towels, no drapes, no instruments."[49] Esther Herman gave birth to her third child, Elana, in her Takoma Park home in March of 1967 with Brew in attendance. "In hospitals I have been draped, strapped down, drugged and made sterile to mention a few of the dehumanizing procedures. At home I was surrounded by bright colors, living plants, my family and affection."[50] The soft spoken Brew was popular with the emerging community of midwives. "He had this aura about him," recalls Ventre. "He reminded me of Jimmy Stewart."[51]

Of course these obstetricians were in the minority, and when they were mentioned in the press, it was seldom in a good light. "Rare is the Area Doctor Who Does Home Deliveries," pronounced Sheila Kast in her article's headline in the *Washington Star-News* on December 2, 1974. Brew and DeVocht, she noted, were on "the minority end of a burning question in the obstetrical community: Do the psychological advantages of giving and receiving birth in warm, familiar surroundings outweigh the added medical risk of not having hospital equipment at hand?" Natural childbirth advocate Dr. Meek offered a clear answer: "NEVER!"[52] Brew and DeVocht were not given the opportunity to defend their position; only to describe the hostility they felt from other obstetricians. Framed this way, there was no chance that the article would present both sides of the issue.

Esther Herman responded in a letter to the editor of the *Washington Star-News* that was published a few weeks later. What about the women who were choosing to give birth at home, she wanted to know. Where was their perspective? "We are the ones the midwives and doctors are servicing, and we would like our feelings known," she wrote. "In general we are an intelligent group of women who want to govern our own bodies. We want our bodies free as we experience the bringing of precious life into this turbulent world." Perhaps more significantly, the assumption that home births were riskier was unsubstantiated, she claimed. Dr. DeLee had made the opposite claim just decades earlier. As Herman put it, "the fact that home deliveries are more risky is just conjecture. There are no solid facts, since none in the medical profession is willing to take on a controlled study."[53]

As the practice of home birth in D.C. increased by the mid-1970s— and perhaps more importantly, became known as a white middle-class phenomenon—the opposition increasingly focused on the question of risk. "Controversial Home Deliveries Rising," stated a 1974 headline in the *Alexandria Gazette*, noting that the "home delivery controversy" was growing in intensity "as the number of home birth adherents steadily increase."[54] Why would women who could afford the safety of a hospital birth opt not to have one? According to a *Washington Post* article, only about 100–150 women chose a home birth in 1974 (based on estimates by doctors and midwives; numbers were undoubtedly higher, as some would have feared legal action). But nearly all of them were white and college educated. "A lot of them are very respectable middle-class people like myself," stated Ventre.[55]

But, the media continued to ask, just how safe was home birth? One reporter noted in 1976, "the subject generates great passion among obstetricians. Perhaps 999 out of every 1,000 totally reject the arguments of the home birth faction, believing that there is always risk to the mother and baby if they do not have the facilities of the modern hospital immediately available." The reporter was able to quote one of the most prominent Washington obstetricians, Dr. John Walsh (Jackie Kennedy's obstetrician), as saying, "I wouldn't do it for a million dollars."[56]

Despite the hype, such controversy was often overstated, proponents believed. "Sure, a hospital is safer," admitted Dr. James Brew. "A train is safer than a car. But I drive." Life was full of risks.[57] Even if Dr. Walsh wouldn't do a home birth for a million dollars, he had colleagues who would. Walsh shared an office with another obstetrician, Dr. Lowell Schwab, in the affluent suburb of Chevy Chase, Maryland. Both were professors at Georgetown University Medical School (along with Dr. Brew). Unlike Walsh, Schwab was extremely supportive of home birth and of the newly emerging midwives. He would regularly refer his clients to Ventre when they were in search of childbirth education. He would also later provide backup for Ventre and other midwives if they needed to transport a home birth client to the hospital. "I would go to his office sometimes with somebody," Ventre recalls, "and you would see all the hippy dippies and then the ladies with white gloves from Chevy Chase or Foxhall Road or McLean."[58] There may have been cultural differences between the clientele, but they were both bringing in much needed revenue. "He got into trouble with Walsh, but you know he brought in a lot of clients, he brought in a lot of women."[59]

FROM BIRTH EDUCATORS TO MIDWIVES

Perhaps the real issue was not where babies were born, but who was attending them. An obstetrician had the training, experience, licensure, and, typically, hospital privileges, which would ensure any emergency transfer would go as smoothly as possible. But D.C. in the 1970s was a far cry from Chicago in the 1950s, and lacked the equivalent of the Chicago Maternity Center. Obstetricians were busy training and practicing at places like the Washington Hospital Center and D.C. General Hospital. Nationwide, their numbers were also shrinking. Dr. J. Robert Willson, President of the American College of Obstetricians and Gynecologists, noted in 1970 that "at least fifteen percent of residency positions are unfilled and more than one-third of the residents on duty are graduates of foreign schools." At this rate, according to obstetrician Dr. Louis Hellman, four out of every ten American babies "will be delivered without a physician of any kind in attendance."[60] The solution, according to Dorothea Lang, director of the Nurse-Midwifery Service Program at the New York City Department of Health, was to replace them with nurse-midwives. "Though the term 'midwife' is apt to conjure up visions of stooped grannies with no formal training, today's certified nurse-midwife is a medically competent professional, up-to-date in every way."[61] She would be the logical alternative.[62]

Lang was not alone in her belief that nurse-midwives could fill the gap. In 1971, ACOG, ACNM, and NAACOG (Nurses Association of the American College of Obstetricians and Gynecologists) approved a "Joint Statement on Maternity Care," marking the first time ACOG recognized nurse-midwifery as a legitimate health profession. The statement called for the "cooperative efforts" of nurses, nurse-midwives, and other personnel working under the direction of obstetricians.[63]

Practical though the solution might be, it did not fit the realities of many areas. Though by the mid-1950s, there were enough nurses identifying as nurse-midwives (approximately 400) to form a national professional organization (the American College of Nurse-Midwives), almost none of them were actually involved in the practice of midwifery, instead working as nursing educators, administrators, or consultants.[64] By the end of the 1960s, there were a mere seven nurse-midwifery education programs across the United States. By 1979, there were a total of nineteen such programs. However, these were programs geared toward hospital deliveries, not home births. Only 8 percent of certified nurse-midwives practicing in 1976–1977 were involved in home births.[65] Many of those most interested in choosing an out-of-hospital birth in the 1970s viewed nurse-midwives as being "complicit with the medical model of childbirth," based on their training and practice under obstetricians.[66]

In the 1970s, Washington D.C. had only a handful of nurse-midwives, primarily because no programs offered the training for these credentials until Georgetown University began a program in 1974. Initially, informal hands-on training took place primarily between lay midwives, childbirth educators, and a handful of physicians. "I went to my first home birth with Phyllis [Stein] at the helm," remembers Alice Bailes. "And she had guts. The baby came out and everything was just fine." Bailes had done plenty of reading on the subject of home birth, but had never actually seen one. One of the students in her childbirth education class asked her to attend her home birth, where she met Dr. DeVocht. Soon she began assisting him. "And that was, you know, when I really learned to have a lot of confidence," she claims.[67] But, she stressed, it was "all very informal." They had to make it up as they were going along. "As there existed no formal structure for our education, we created our own."[68]

Often the home birth doctors took responsibility. Dr. James Brew, referred to by one journalist as "the daddy of home births," was pivotal in the training of these self-proclaimed lay midwives.[69] "My wish for the near future is that there would be more midwives working," he said in 1976. "This would get the word out and circumvent the doctors who are unwilling to deliver at home."[70] By that year, he claimed to have delivered around 550 babies at home over the past twenty years. "The demand," he said, "was always more than I could handle."[71]

Not all of Brew's trainees identified as lay midwives. Jan Epstein and Marion McCartney worked for Brew as nurses before opening a home birth practice together, with Brew serving as emergency backup. "That's how I got started doing home births," Epstein explained in a 1981 interview. Brew was "being inundated with requests for home delivery. He couldn't handle all of them. Soon he said to me, 'Jan, why don't you go to midwifery school and then you can do the home births. Then I don't have to be there."[72] McCartney and Epstein, like Ventre, would practice as home certified nurse-midwives after graduating from the Georgetown program.

While practicing, Brew did not always make it to births on time. He had a reputation for waiting until the last minute, which often was too late. When Esther Herman gave birth to her fourth child, David, in July of 1973, Brew was still in surgery and missed the delivery. Phyllis Stein caught the baby with Fran Ventre at her side. "What I witnessed that day transformed my entire conception of birth," Ventre wrote. "The skill, sensitivity, and caring of one woman for another in helping her at this crucial time to gently give birth to her child was a very powerful and moving experience for me."[73] Stein remembers it as a very peaceful, easy birth.[74]

Ventre later claimed that she made the decision to go into midwifery based on Herman's birth. "I realized that this midwife [Stein] was practicing a beautiful art, one that I had never experienced with an obstetrician in the hospital." Brew wasn't needed. They could do it on their own, she realized, and so committed herself to joining the underground network. "The physicians felt their presence was no longer necessary at the births," explained Alice Bailes. Gradually, we realized we had a name. We began calling ourselves 'lay midwives'."[75]

More and more couples either contacted these lay midwives directly or were referred to them by DeVocht and Brew. Gene Declercq and his wife Carol were expecting their second child in 1975 and, after interviewing DeVocht, who had come "highly recommended," they decided to do a home birth. DeVocht suggested they also select a lay midwife to assist him at the birth. Declercq recalls that DeVocht was "probably a little condescending" about the midwives, stressing that they made very good supporters, rather than actual practitioners. "But he was so matter of fact about all of it." They started going to H.O.M.E. meetings, where they met Ventre and her associate, Tina Long, whom they chose to assist DeVocht at the birth.[76]

Eventually, DeVocht recognized that women like Long and Bailes were needed as more than just assistants at home births. Bailes remembers how she transitioned from assistant to midwife. "One day," she recalls, "one of my students called me and said, 'Dr. DeVocht told me that you would help me have my baby at home'. And I said, 'No, no, no. He meant that I would help him help you have your baby at home.' And she said, 'No, he wouldn't be available. He's gotten too busy'. .. so my first primary birth was with my 9-week-old son on my back and Fran [Ventre] next to me."

Suddenly finding themselves in charge, many of these women came under increased scrutiny, particularly when things went wrong. In June of 1974, Ventre's colleague, Tina Long, was threatened with arrest for practicing medicine without a license in the state of Virginia. One of her mothers had suffered a second-degree tear when the baby's shoulder first emerged and had to go to the hospital for stitches. A vice squad detective followed this mother's case and threatened to arrest Long if she did not sign a document promising to never again practice midwifery. Getting licensed was no easy task; Long had attempted to apply the previous year in the state of Virginia, but legal loopholes made it impossible.

"LAY" VERSUS NURSE-MIDWIFE: THE HIERARCHY OF LICENSURE

Ventre vowed not to suffer the same penalty. She contacted health officials in Montgomery County, Maryland to inquire about lay licensure and was told that no one had applied since 1924. Nonetheless, she obtained an application and provided evidence of assisting at forty births, along with character statements. She believed that her experience and reputation demonstrated her qualifications for licensure.

State and county officials disagreed. County Health Officer Dr. Lindgren wrote that he would prefer to see nurse-midwives assist home births. "If [nurse-midwives] are not available and the alternative is between trained lay midwives and husbands, I would opt for the lay midwives." This was hardly a ringing endorsement. The key was to make sure they were supervised by doctors. "I would not like to see midwives in this county, no matter how well-trained, unless they are working in close association with physicians."[77] Months passed, and when pressed again, Lindgren declared that he had no intention of licensing lay midwives and that it was not his responsibility to deal with the application.

Ventre then learned from another source that, as the result of her application, the Maryland State Board of Health was attempting to repeal the law sanctioning the use of lay midwives. She had two days to prepare a statement if she wanted to try to prevent the repeal. She panicked as she thought about her full day of college physiology lab, her husband out of town, her three children at home, and a Lamaze class to teach in the evening. "I felt overwhelmed. There was so little time and so much at stake," she recalled. On the day of the hearing, she worked until 5 a.m. on the statement, typed it up, and went to bed. Two hours later, she got up, took her children to school, and drove to Annapolis. "It was a clear spring-like day and I felt a surge of confidence," she remembered. "If I lost the battle, I would at least have tried."[78]

Nothing prepared her for the shock she encountered upon entering the Senate building for the hearing. When she signed her name at the entrance, she discovered a slew of names ahead of hers, many of them certified nurse-midwives working for the Public Health Service. Suddenly she realized that it was her application that had generated the movement to repeal the midwifery law and that many nurse-midwives were part of the opposition.

Why weren't they on the same side? Though relations in the D.C. area between the certified nurse-midwives and the lay midwives had been relatively benign and, indeed, often mutually supportive, Ventre's application had become a sticking point. As would become increasingly clear in the late 1970s and 1980s, the question of education, certification, and licensure would divide not only midwives and obstetricians, but also different types of midwives. A clear hierarchy existed, even at the point of licensure. As one midwife wrote of this time period, certified nurse-midwives often "rejected apprentice midwifery as inferior and midwives who entered the practice of midwifery through this route as endangering the health and safety of women and children."[79] Being called upon to catch a baby or two when the doctor didn't show up on time, or helping friends deliver at home, they believed, did not entitle these women to call themselves licensed midwives or to see themselves as equals in the birthing room.

Ventre anxiously sat in the corner of the hearing room of the Economic Affairs Committee. Then her small group of supporters arrived—one pregnant, one nursing an infant, and another with a toddler, physical reminders of the nature of the debate. Ventre's confidence increased when the committee chairman noted that he had been born at home, delivered by a granny midwife.

When the chairman called her name, she nervously approached the podium, noting the surprised reactions of the public health midwives and health officials who had assumed she would not learn of the hearing. She knew what she needed to say and how to contextualize this debate. She explained the origins of the natural childbirth movement and the growing dissatisfaction of American women with hospital births. She compared maternal and infant mortality rates of the United States with countries who routinely utilized home births to argue that it was in fact safer to give birth at home than in the hospital. And she stressed the inevitable trend toward home births, urging the committee to allow experienced lay midwives to ensure the safety of such a trend.

Her testimony proved influential. Much to Ventre's relief, the committee allowed the law to remain on the books. Her positive impression on the committee elicited one Senator's own home birth story in the lobby after the hearing, followed by his assurance that the law was safe.[80]

But the battle was not yet won. Only after Ventre's lawyer threatened action against the state, which continued to delay processing her application, did she make headway. She agreed to create a formal training plan, one that included attending more home births along with Dr. Brew. Once this was completed and she passed an examination, she became fully licensed in the state of Maryland. In the fall of 1975, she drove to Rockville to officially register, bribing her children to accompany her by bringing several of their friends along. She arrived, along with her "boisterous entourage," at the Circuit Court to sign her name. "When I opened the dusty old Registry for Lay Midwives, I was moved by the honest names of these old granny midwives before me carefully inscribed in calligraphy," she recalled. Only four names were listed, the first from 1913, the last in 1924. "Here I was, some fifty years later, a continuing link with these dedicated ghosts of the past. . . . I was now one of them."[81]

If licensure was the only thing keeping Ventre from practicing midwifery legally in the state of Maryland, her struggle would have ended on that day. But the law stipulated that she had to have medical backup in order to practice her trade, and most local obstetricians refused. Without such backup, she could lose her license and possibly face imprisonment. "I have not gone underground again because I feel a strong commitment to keeping this license as it sets a precedent making it possible for other lay midwives to obtain it," she explained.[82]

The only solution, she believed, was to go back to school. With a nursing degree, she could continue on to get a certificate in nurse-midwifery at Georgetown University. Such an education, she believed, would help her expand her knowledge and skills. It would provide her with more opportunities to practice her trade and increase her legitimacy in the eyes of organized medicine. She would also be represented by a professional organization, the ACNM. It would also, however, come at a personal cost, as some of her fellow lay midwives saw such a move as a sign of betrayal.

Nonetheless, if she wanted the support of obstetricians (which, as she had learned, was essential in order to obtain emergency backup), becoming a CNM was a smart move. The local ACOG chapter was well aware of the rise in home births and was eager to reinforce the obstetrician's primary role as birth attendant.[83] But nurse-midwifery was not the real problem, since those practitioners were at least credentialed, licensed, and regulated by a professional nursing organization. Dr. Vince Fitzpatrick, vice-chairman for the Maryland chapter of ACOG, noted that "nurse-midwives and doctors are getting to the point of being on good terms. The term 'collaborate' was agreed upon and represents an equal status between doctors and nurses."[84]

Lay midwives were another matter entirely. They had no professional organization in the 1970s. They often worked underground, aware that what they were doing was illegal (or at least extralegal). One ACOG fellow noted that many lay midwives practicing underground in South Carolina "are apparently being concealed by having the father of the babies sign the birth certificate."[85] Many babies born at home simply didn't have birth certificates, complicating attempts to gather statistics. At least in one case, Ventre did not always file one, even after receiving her lay midwifery license from the state. "We have received a request from the parents of the above named subject for her birth certificate. They have stated that the child was delivered at home by you," wrote the Chief of the Division of Vital Records in the Maryland Department of Health and Mental Hygiene two months after the birth. "As of this date we have not received any birth certificate for this child signed by you," he wrote. He enclosed a self-addressed stamped envelope and a birth certificate for her to return.[86]

As obstetricians and state legislators began to understand the existence of two different types of midwives, most recognized nurse-midwifery as the lesser of two evils and focused their energy on keeping lay midwives out of bedrooms and hospitals. For ACOG, this meant hiring lobbyists in every district to fight against midwifery bills. It meant recruiting mothers who had to be transferred from home to hospital after an emergency situation arose to testify against these bills. It meant rewarding fellows who took a stand against home birth. The 1980 ACOG Wyeth Policy Research Award was given to Dr. Philip Henderson for his proposal, "Lay Midwifery Bill: Operation Democracy." The committee noted that "Dr. Henderson utilized multiple organizations as well as individuals to bring pressure against the Lay Midwifery Bill since he felt it was an inferior piece of legislation."[87] Non-nurse midwives needed to be stopped, and the most effective strategy was through the state legislature. Successful attempts to prevent legislation, or to introduce restrictive legislation, should be studied, disseminated, and rewarded, ACOG believed.

Three years after Ventre testified before the Maryland state senate economic affairs committee to demand her own licensure, she was back to defend the lay midwifery law, again under attack. A new bill had been introduced requiring all midwives who practiced in the state to be licensed by the state as registered nurses as well. Ventre called this requirement "superfluous and restrictive," setting up a "double criterion for one set of practitioners which is not required of other professionals." What the authors of the bill did not seem to understand, she argued, was that lay midwives came from a different background. "I would like to clarify to this committee the difference between the lay midwife and the certified nurse-midwife," she began. Whereas the CNM came from a background in nursing, the lay midwife "usually started out as a vocal consumer of maternity care." She typically began as a childbirth educator working to change the hospital maternity environment. But "as the home birth phenomenon gained momentum in this state and nationally we were called upon to assist those couples who having made the decision to give birth at home found themselves abandoned by the medical profession." People like Ventre, Bailes, Long, and Stein became midwives "not because we had actively chosen this as a profession but because we were willing to take on the responsibility. We empathized with the home-oriented couples and desperately wanted to see a need filled that the physician <u>would not fill</u> and the nurse-midwife <u>could not fill</u>."[88]

The problem was not the lay midwives, Ventre countered. It was the fact that the "established medical community has denigrated them" and denied them training and licensure. "For the sake of consumer protection, a viable, updated law regulating standards of practice for midwives in today's maternity care is obviously imperative." But the proposed law excluded them. "If this law allows for the licensing of only *nurse*-midwives, it will not necessarily stop the lay midwives. They will continue to practice in growing numbers, as they do nationwide, outside of the law and the state will have no regulatory mechanism to monitor standards or assure its citizens of minimum competence." [89] Ventre's passionate testimony failed to convince the committee. It would be more than thirty years before Maryland would again license non-nurse midwives; HB 9 legalizing non-nurse midwives attending home births passed in May of 2015.[90] As delegate Ariana Kelly, who sponsored HB 9, noted, "medical licensing bills are brutal. They're turf wars."[91] That much had not changed over the decades.

BACK TO SCHOOL: MONTGOMERY COLLEGE AND GEORGETOWN UNIVERSITY

Ventre wrote her testimony while attending nursing school at Montgomery College, well aware that without such a degree it would be virtually impossible to continue to practice midwifery legally—despite the fact that she was licensed. She recognized that she had personally lost the battle for alternative training and licensure of non-nurse midwives even as she kept up the fight. As a result, she found nursing school exceedingly frustrating. It was challenging to commit herself to the study of topics that she did not believe would enhance her career as a midwife. "I am aware of some of the important elements in nurse's training to the practice of midwifery," she explained to the state senate committee. "I also recognize that alternate backgrounds and experiences likewise provide important elements crucial to midwifery. But, I do not recognize the heavy emphasis in caring for orthopedic patients, hernia patients, heart attack victims and cancer patients as adding to one's ability to qualify for accredited midwifery."[92]

Associate degree programs in nursing, offered at community colleges, grew from seven in the 1950s to nearly 700 by the time Ventre enrolled at Montgomery.[93] Previously, the nursing profession required a four-year bachelor's degree program. "They were out to prove that community college nursing programs could do as well," Ventre explained. "And so in doing that they were very hard on us . . . every year it was very important that when we took the nursing boards that we got higher than anyone in this state."[94]

At Montgomery College, Ventre studied obstetrical nursing with a former Catholic nun, Irene Morelli. On Ventre's first day of class, Morelli lectured on natural childbirth and how it worked. She then stopped, mid-sentence: "'I won't say anymore because there are some childbirth educators—one of whom is in this class—who are very adamant and would make women feel guilty'," Ventre remembers her saying. "And I thought, is she talking about me?" After the break some classmates congratulated Ventre on keeping her mouth shut.[95] Her loud voice and distinct Brooklyn accent, combined with her outspoken passion for natural childbirth, meant that her reputation preceded her.

It was not obstetrical nursing that Ventre found most relevant to her career path as a midwife, but psychiatric nursing, taught by nursing professor Eunice Crisan. What she witnessed during her fifteen-week clinical at St. Elizabeths Hospital, which provided the majority of inpatient psychiatric services in the District of Columbia at the time, fundamentally challenged the way she understood pain. Though she herself expressed frustration at the course requirements seemingly unrelated to maternity care, her experience with male psychiatric patients ultimately helped her rethink how to help laboring women process the pain and fear of childbirth. Therapeutic techniques for emotional distress, she realized, could apply to childbirth as well.

Located on a plateau above the Anacostia River in Southeast Washington, St. Elizabeths opened its doors in 1855 as the Government Hospital for the Insane and went from being celebrated as a model asylum in the nineteenth century to being derided for mismanagement, overcrowding, and mistreatment in the twentieth.[96] When Ventre was working there, St. Elizabeths housed 2,200 patients and was in the midst of turmoil.[97] The hospital had recently lost its accreditation from the Joint Commission on Accreditation of Hospitals due to its failure to meet certain standards, including overcrowding and a lack of therapeutic counseling.[98] In response, the hospital increased personnel in nursing, social work, psychology, and therapy. But psychological services, according to a governmental report in 1977, were "still not provided in some wards on a regular basis." Management appeared to be "reactive and crisis oriented." Little had been done to meet patients' therapeutic needs, in part because "all clinical staff spend much time attending meetings and thus away from patients."[99]

Ventre documented her experience through "reaction logs" assigned by Professor Crisan. The logs reflect this tumultuous time in the hospital's history as well as her own fears, struggles, and insights. "I can't deny that I came to St. Elizabeth's reluctantly," she wrote on January 29, 1976.[100] "I felt some of the youthful idealism reawaken," she wrote, when meeting the staff for the first time. "They were in the throes of tragedy, the violent death of a fellow staff member committed by a patient. I sat there in awe of their stamina and ability to deal 'straight' with their own emotions and their fellow workers. They not only have learned the art of survival of such a place but I could see that they would grow together and stronger from it. There was no room here for phony emotions or sentiments."[101] After years of involvement in the intensity and drama of birth, she found some value in processing the equally intense realities of death.

Although initially she did not see a connection between psychiatric nursing and midwifery, what she gained in those few months influenced her future career as a midwife. She began to formulate connections between all types of suffering, whether physical, emotional, or spiritual. Professor Crisan encouraged her to focus on the connections and overlaps between midwifery and psychiatric nursing. "They both go together," she wrote in the margins of Ventre's reaction log. They "supplement each other."[102] Ventre agreed. "This experience is helping me in relating more effectively with the people I deal with in my own area. I'm becoming a little more aware of my own feelings and needs in these relationships and how I can use or separate them from the needs of the couples coming to my classes."[103]

Ventre, along with her three fellow nursing students, was assigned to Ward 12, an all-male maximum security ward in the John Howard Pavilion. The Pavilion housed all of St. Elizabeths' forensic patients—those committed after being found not guilty of a crime by reason of insanity (such as its most infamous patient, John Hinckley, Jr.). They represented 11 percent of the total patient population at the hospital.[104] Almost all of the men in Ward 12 were African American, reflecting the hospital's patient population, which was disproportionately black and poor.[105] The patients and surrounding neighborhood was culturally foreign to Ventre's experience in affluent, white Chevy Chase, Maryland.

Ventre found the all-black staff on the ward to be "outstanding," crediting the supervisor, Mr. Jones. "Employee morale appears to be higher and that, I believe is a credit to Mr. Jones and his respect of their ability."[106] Ventre described Jones as "charismatic," noting, "if I were a psychiatric nurse I would work at St. Elizabeth's only because of him."[107] He helped her to begin to understand the powerful presence of racism in the hospital and D.C. more generally.

Therapy at St. Elizabeths was anything but conventional. Each day started off with dance therapy, which Ventre explained as a process that "allows for free expression and body movement as a nonverbal form of communication to help the patients release tension, anger or feelings which may be difficult to express verbally."[108] As a former Lamaze coach, Ventre could identify with the notion that physical movement, whether in the form of heavy breathing or dance moves, could release tension. The leaders of the dance therapy program at St. Elizabeths emphasized its role as a "psychotherapeutic tool" to "develop a more viable body image ... sense of self and one's power to control one's life, movement fundamentals and grow locomotion patterns." Their most basic goal was the development of "body awareness, body efficiency, body image and a sense of oneself."[109]

Dance therapy as practiced at St. Elizabeths was intended to reorient the relationship between the physical body and human emotion. Home birth midwives, of course, advocated a similar position. Medicated birth prevented a laboring woman from physically experiencing the birth of her child, they believed; numbing the pain came at the expense of maternal infant bonding. Ventre witnessed this similarity firsthand when she danced alongside the patients of Ward 12. "At the beginning everyone expressed feelings of being tense, self-conscious and fidgety, especially since four new student nurses were involved in the dance therapy," she noted. Over time, she picked up some of the nuances in the patients' movements, the moments of stiffness, the "lack of movement of the torso and shoulders" that "hinted at the problems and difficulties they had with resolving their feelings."[110] Working one on one with patient "Mr. M," she noticed a change both in his emotional behavior and his physical appearance at the next dance therapy session. "It was as though his body had opened up and had filled out," she wrote triumphantly.[111]

Dance therapy offered the men of Ward 12 the opportunity to do what most non-institutionalized residents of D.C. could not—have guided conversations between blacks and whites about racism. Other forms of therapy elicited conversations about relationships and family. Mr. Jones discussed "components of courtship and how family living experience influences the ability to have a meaningful relationship with someone of the opposite sex." Poor familial relationships in early childhood inhibited future relationships, he explained. Ventre noted that Jones "elicited much response from the men themselves to reach these conclusions." He also used role playing to "demonstrate a courtship procedure," where the patients had to offer advice about what a man and woman should say to each other when courting.[112]

Jones' lecture served as a preparatory session for a presentation Ventre gave the following week on "natural childbirth and the family experience" at the suggestion of her teacher Mrs. Crisan. "There were many nice comments regarding your lecture," Crisan noted in the margins of Ventre's journal afterwards. Ventre was pleased at how well it went, particularly the level of patient participation. "I was glad that they did get involved and seemed genuinely interested as I have always taught these classes to the white middle class and didn't think I could relate to this segment of the population," she wrote.[113] She delivered the lecture a second time for another ward, but found it to be more awkward with a group she had never met before. It is hard to even imagine the setup: a young white middle-class activist childbirth educator and midwife lecturing about natural childbirth to a group of African American men labeled criminally insane. The reaction was not as enthusiastic as in Ward 12, she noted, but many came up to her afterwards to ask personal questions or to "discuss things that they didn't feel comfortable with in the group discussion."[114]

Ventre's clinical experience at St. Elizabeths enabled her to see her role as a midwife and educator from a psychological perspective. In her final report for Mrs. Crisan, she developed a "Parent Education Course Design," structured similarly to what she was already teaching at home as part of her new organization, Home Oriented Maternity Experience. She defined her role as one that would "strengthen patients' inner resources." "A teacher who is sensitive to the needs of the couples gives them the tools to realize their own strengths in coping with the demands of labor and delivery," she explained. "S/he does not foster a dependency relationship, but rather, helps them attain their own potential and ability to function independently." Ventre continued, "as individuals deeply committed to 'prepared, natural childbirth, we have strong values, but a responsibility not to impose our values upon the members of the class. A non-judgmental attitude of the instructor helps assure them that their concerns or fears have validity and that it's okay to express them." Crisan circled "non-judgmental," writing in the margins: "Yes! See me about this. You are one of the first to truly define this well."[115] This exchange on paper continued in person. Thirty-five years later, Ventre recounted the significance of Crisan's comments:

> She taught me a great lesson. Because there are certain things that I said or maybe wrote that might have been controversial. And when she advised me she said, 'you know you have a very important future. So you have to be especially careful of what you say. And how you say it. You have a responsibility to be very careful about your words. To understand who your audience is and how they're going to be accepting it. Otherwise you won't be heard.' And it was the best, I mean I couldn't always keep it, being from Brooklyn. But she did it in such a positive way, telling me that I was going to be making

a very big contribution. . . . She was very kind, yet she could give me a criticism but in a positive way. Where you learned from your mistakes rather than being punished for them. And I always tried as much as possible to remember that.[116]

After completing her RN degree at Montgomery College, Ventre continued her studies in nurse-midwifery at Georgetown University. The nine-month post-baccalaureate program was the first to offer the CNM degree in the D.C. metropolitan area.[117] Establishing such a program in Washington, D.C. was a risky endeavor, because the legal status of midwifery remained uncertain in the district. But the previous spring, the D.C. Medical Society and the District of Columbia Nurses' Association adopted a policy statement "recognizing nurse-midwifery as a specialized area of registered nursing and describing the authority and functions of same."[118] This agreement paved the way for the creation of a local training program.

The Georgetown nurse-midwifery program started in February of 1974 with an incoming class of six "excellent" student nurse-midwives. According to the nurse-midwifery faculty, "favorable publicity" resulted in a high number of highly qualified applicants, and the selected admits were "composed of highly motivated individuals who are certain to be a credit to their professional field."[119] Courses included "the science of obstetrics," genetics and embryology, nutrition, the anatomy and physiology of reproduction, neonatology, sociological aspects of childbearing and family living, and psychological aspects of childbearing and family living.[120]

Marion McCartney was among the six "highly motivated individuals" to enroll in the first nurse-midwifery class at Georgetown. She had studied nursing at Catholic University, but after graduating, focused on marriage, motherhood, and teaching childbirth education. Then suddenly, she recalls, the Georgetown program opened up. "So I said to my husband, 'I really want to do this.' And he said, 'oh it won't be that bad.' I said, 'it's going to be very time consuming.' He said, 'I don't know—graduate school isn't *that* difficult.' And I was like, 'well, this is really not like an ordinary graduate school.'"[121]

McCartney discovered not only that she was competent but that there were disparities in teaching techniques between nurse-midwifery and obstetric medicine. Several of the required courses in the curriculum were taught by and for the medical school. "The doctors believed that if we were up against the medical students we would flunk out and that would be the end of the program," she theorized. Instead, the handful of nurse-midwife students aced the classes. "They weren't that hard." She had already studied OB/GYN at Catholic University with a nurse-midwife who was a major proponent of natural childbirth. "She was really into it," recalled McCartney,

"I could see it work over and over again." This experience had inspired her to be a childbirth educator. When taking her CNM classes, she discovered that she had much more experience than the medical students. "These guys didn't know how to do a vaginal exam, they didn't know the difference between effacement and dilatation, but they knew all this esoteric stuff that they'd never see in their lives."[122]

The problem was not just with the medical students but with the style of teaching. "Our lectures in nursing school were so much better than what I was listening to," she said. Different doctors rotated in to teach various sections of a class. "But nobody taught the basics. Nobody was saying, 'this is what a normal delivery looks like.' They had no idea." Medical students, she realized, were trained very differently than nurses. "Their method of teaching clinical was to give very little information and then scream at them if they made a mistake. And that was kind of like being in the military. It was awful."[123] Like many midwives, McCartney valued hands-on experience, just as Joseph DeLee had decades before. Her concern was similar to what his had been—the lack of opportunity to attend a hospital birth. "It was very hard to get deliveries," she explained. D.C. General was the primary teaching hospital. The student nurse-midwives competed for spots to train there with medical students from Georgetown and Howard Universities. "Everybody wanted to do deliveries there." She would sometimes sneak into Georgetown Hospital to observe a delivery with Dr. Brew, though the obstetricians were often infuriated by her presence. "I just knew I could learn so much by just watching and watching and watching and asking questions."[124]

Proponents of nurse-midwifery training programs found themselves in the same conundrum DeLee had been in fifty years earlier. In order to promote their profession, they had to provide clinical experience for their students. Nurse-midwives needed exposure to the delivery room, yet were met with resistance by many in the obstetrical profession. As the creators of the Georgetown nurse-midwifery program noted in their first-year self-evaluation, "the principal weakness lies in the ambivalent attitude of professionals in the health field toward the nurse-midwife. Much remains to be done to convince such professionals to accept the nurse-midwife as a member of the health care team." Professional acceptance was "crucial to the development of nurse-midwifery services within the health care facilities of the Washington, D.C. area and of clinical sites which would provide students with the desired number of cases."[125]

Even those nurse-midwives who would go on to practice in out-of-hospital settings needed hospital births in order to become certified. They faced the same problems as DeLee did, but in reverse. Under DeLee's plan, medical students needed the home experience to do hospital births, while nurse-midwifery students needed the hospital experience in order to do home births.

The solution in both cases rested with a similar client base: poor, inner-city African Americans. In Chicago, it was the Chicago Maternity Center. In the District of Columbia, it was D.C. General, the city's first and only public hospital. In the 1970s, it suffered similar problems to St. Elizabeths: poor conditions, lack of funds, overcrowding, and understaffing. "Everybody agreed that care was inadequate," remembered Martin Shargel who finished his residency at D.C. General from 1968 to 1971. "Everybody agreed that there was overcrowding, everybody agreed that there wasn't enough money."[126] Located next to the D.C. jail, it was, like Chicago's Cook County Hospital, a place to avoid if at all possible. Patients were those who could not afford to go elsewhere, and in a city that was 72 percent black in 1970, that meant they were nearly all African American and poor.

Not unrelated, Washington D.C. also suffered from alarmingly high infant mortality and morbidity rates. According to the Mayor's Task Force on Public Health Goals, D.C. ranked second only to the state of Mississippi in infant mortality in 1970.[127] Thus the pilot nurse-midwifery program at D.C. General launched in 1974 was aimed at improving the abysmal local infant mortality rates and providing training for certified nurse-midwives.

Within a year, the Service proved somewhat successful in assuaging doubts about the use of nurse-midwives. Patients seemed to appreciate the more "comprehensive family centered maternity care" in which they could see the same midwife from their first prenatal appointment through their six-week postpartum visit. "The greatest gratification I have experienced is that patients have requested Nurse-Midwifery Service care in lieu of care by the physician," wrote the director of the service, "after having talked with other patients who have been under our care." She noted an "initial wariness" from the medical staff, followed by "their expression of their desire for the services of Nurse-Midwives in their personal and professional experiences." Within the first thirteen months, nurse-midwives supervised a total of fifty-four births (assisted by the handful of Georgetown student nurse-midwives) at D.C. General.[128]

The pilot project was not without problems. Funding was a "constant struggle." There had been "unanticipated communication breakdowns" between the director of the Georgetown School of Nursing, the Department of Human Resources, and the nurse-midwifery program.[129] While some of the hospital staff may have welcomed the additional help, not all obstetricians would have been pleased that some of their patients, when given the choice, preferred nurse-midwives over physicians for their maternity care.

By the fall of 1975, twelve students had gone through the nurse-midwifery program at Georgetown and become certified nurse-midwives.

Fran Ventre, Alice Bailes, and Marsha Jackson would follow a few years later. Yet despite the decline in OB/GYN residency applications—and therefore the need for an alternative type of birth practitioner—most local hospitals were not yet comfortable with hiring nurse-midwives. The nurse-midwifery service at D.C. General did not become the new model. "There were no jobs for midwives," recalled Jan Epstein, who graduated the program in 1975.[130]

FROM HOSPITAL TO HOME

After graduating from Georgetown and becoming licensed CNMs, Ventre, Epstein, McCartney, Bailes, and Jackson all returned to the business of out-of-hospital births. Eventually, they would all become involved in running birth centers. In the meantime, they focused on delivering babies at home, and developing the business structure and organization that would make such a practice sustainable.

Clients expressed appreciation for the opportunity to have a home birth with a midwife. "I wanted to thank you for making my birth experience one that I will remember and cherish for years to come," wrote one of Ventre's clients. "You really made this experience very special, working with me to help the contractions and pushes, being very supportive, [and] giving great suggestions." What made the birth special was not only the sense of support, but also trust. "I can't thank you enough for your knowledge, expertise, support, and experience in bringing my child into this world," she declared.[131] "You were so calm and gentle," wrote another client.[132] A third added how much her husband felt involved in the birth "because you made him feel that way. It was a great experience for both of us because you truly made us feel in control."[133]

While Ventre worked independently, Epstein and McCartney created their own business, the first certified nurse-midwife practice in the area. Both had assisted Dr. Brew at home births prior to obtaining their degrees. Once certified, they took over his practice and he served as emergency backup. They formed a corporation, Maternity Center Associates, and rented office space across the street from Brew in a newly constructed medical office building in Bethesda. In addition to Brew's referrals, their clientele learned about them through word of mouth, newspaper and magazine articles, La Leche League groups, and childbirth education groups.

By 1981, Maternity Center Associates were doing somewhere between 250 and 300 home births per year, and their staff had grown.[134] Esther Herman conducted breastfeeding and child development courses for them from 1977 to 1981. Barbara Vaughey joined the practice as a third midwife, as demand for their services grew. Marsha Jackson worked with them as a birth assistant before she attended Georgetown and became a nurse-midwife. Jackson recalls that the Center "always made a point to refer their Black clients to me for birth assistant services. We would usually figure out during the phone call that we were both Black. Clients would laugh, but appreciated when they figured out that they were steered to me because of our ethnic sisterhood."[135]

The majority of their clients were white. "We really had a very middle class, upper middle-class clientele," explained McCartney. "I mean it was *Bethesda*." This was not the same type of client as she saw at D.C. General or that Jackson would see as she became involved at Howard University Hospital. "And they were the people who read, you know? They were looking for something different," McCartney continued. "And a lot of them were nurses who'd come to us. Who'd worked labor and delivery. And they didn't want to do it that way. And they knew they didn't have a snowball's chance if they went into the hospital to control anything because if you're in the hospital, that's it."[136]

Many D.C. area residents learned about Epstein and McCartney's business in the local newspaper. Colorful stories and vivid photographs captured the growing practice of these no-nonsense midwives. One story in the *Washington Star* described McCartney as "a tiny woman in cord trousers and a sweater" who "seemed to stay detached from the joy and the sweat in the room."[137] McCartney later reflected, "You know, we were very careful about how we dressed and what we said." Epstein agreed. "We tried to be in the mainstream. Not mainstream, but *in* it. So that, you know, there would be some recognition that way. They wouldn't see us as kooks out there somewhere."[138]

Birth stories covered by the media also helped establish home birth as a not-so-radical middle-class practice in the D.C. area. NBC News correspondent Douglas Kiker watched his second child born at home under the care of McCartney and Brew. He was initially "violently opposed to the idea," and threatened to run away to the nearby Zebra Room, a popular local bar and pizza joint in Northwest Washington. But he relented, and the experience turned him into a convert. He wrote an essay on the topic which received "an enormous response from all over the country." He characterized home birth as "not at all messy," "absolutely thrilling," nothing to be afraid of, and very cheap. He estimated that his son's birth had cost them $350. "It's a white, middle class trend but I suspect that a lot of women all over the country are deeply interested in the subject."[139]

To be sure, Epstein and McCartney had their share of eclectic cases. Epstein remembers one client who lived with a menagerie of snakes, lizards and birds. "I happened to not like snakes and birds. Lizards, you know, they were in a tank, I didn't think they'd be a problem," she continued. "But it smelled so bad that I finally put my bag down, I checked her, and I said, 'we can't deliver here. We have to deliver in a hospital.'"[140] When an assistant would visit a client's home prior to a delivery, she would assess the cleanliness of the home on a scale of one to ten if Epstein was the midwife on call. She disliked delivering in a dirty house.

McCartney also emphasized cleanliness and a safe and hygienic delivery. She remembers a client living in Virginia whose house was crowded with drug paraphernalia and lots of people. "I thought oh my god I hadn't seen that many drugs ever in my life. I mean there was pot everywhere. And then there were these little glassine things and I thought 'I don't even want to know what's in those. Just get those out of the house.' I want a clean house. I don't want any illegal substances."[141] Upholding their solid reputation was crucial.

Durrin films provided McCartney with a powerful way to convey her reputation. On September 20, 1981, PBS aired *Daughters of Time*, a thirty-minute documentary contracted by ASPO. It was the first film that "was talking about midwifery for the middle class, not as only an option for the poor. So it was really exciting; midwives were very excited."[142] The film, which was a finalist in the American Film Festival, featured three certified nurse-midwives (Sister Angela Murdaugh, Linda Viera, and Marion McCartney) in three different settings: a freestanding birth center in Texas, a hospital in Colorado, and a home birth in suburban Maryland. As La Leche League founder Marian Tompson declared, "At last, a film which takes the mystery out of midwifery."[143] McCartney delivers the baby at home in the final moments of the film. Viewers also see her testifying before Congress alongside Congressman Al Gore, cheering at her daughter's soccer game, teaching a class, driving her suburban station wagon, and examining pregnant patients at her birth center. She is a lobbyist, teacher, birth practitioner, and mom. She is well coiffed, stylish, youthful, and good looking—the poster child of the modern nurse-midwife.

THE MIDDLE-CLASS MIDWIFE

By 1981, when *Daughters of Time* aired, the American College of Nurse-Midwives strongly believed that promoting nurse-midwifery as safe and modern was crucial to stabilizing their place in maternity care. Their numbers had increased dramatically in the past quarter-century; there were now over 2,000 nurse-midwives in the United States, approximately 1,200 of whom were delivering babies. They were gradually being accepted in hospitals, first to care for the poor but increasingly for the middle class.[144]

Establishing a reputation as a responsible, middle-class profession, they believed, would solidify their client base at a time when consumers were shopping for providers with whom they could identify.

Changes in birth practices had not and would not come from the medical or nursing professions, McCartney explained in *Daughters of Time*, but from the consumer. Prospective parents, shopping for birth providers, should be well aware of what nurse-midwives and out-of-hospital birth had to offer. "For a long time I would go to deliveries and arrive at the door and the parents of the woman in labor would be at the birth and they would open the door and say oh, I really was expecting someone totally different looking," McCartney says in the film, while driving to a home delivery.[145] Ideally, a widely viewed film like *Daughters of Time* would educate consumers and popularize the profession, not just as a safety valve to combat high infant mortality in inner-city hospitals, but as a middle-class ideal. "It was not a hippie thing," Fran Ventre insisted later.[146] Home birth was not, as assumed, "a phenomenon of the hippies and the counterculture," wrote her friend Esther Herman.[147]

And yet, some mothers seeking an alternative birth viewed nurse-midwives with suspicion, believing they were "complicit with the medical model of childbirth."[148] They found the philosophy and apprenticeship training of the lay midwife far more appealing and the one most likely to produce a meaningful birth experience. As a result, nurse-midwives faced competition both from the more medically oriented obstetrician and the more spiritually oriented lay midwife.

CHAPTER 3

✿

Psychedelic Birth

The Emergence of the Hippie Midwife

On the West Coast, a 1970s home birth was far more likely to occur in a teepee or a commune than a suburban ranch house. While alternative birthers across the country shared some common characteristics, including a general critique of hospital births, those in California tended to blend spirituality with science in their prescription for better birthing. Opting out of the hospital, they believed, heightened the sacred aspects of birth, enhanced the maternal–infant bond, and provided the potential to form a more perfect family union. In this context, childbirth was a catalyst to spiritual transcendence.

At the same time, new developments in psychiatric research and the proliferation of psychoactive substances created a vibrant, albeit surprising, intellectual exchange between hippies, midwives, and some psychiatrists about the meaning and significance of birth. This chapter exposes the resulting unexpected entanglements between psychedelic psychiatry and spiritual midwifery by focusing on the creation of the longest lasting hippie commune, The Farm. Though The Farm was established in Summertown, Tennessee, its founders traveled from San Francisco to build their utopia where farmland was cheaper. They brought with them intellectual and practical tools gathered from as far away as Communist China and Czechoslovakia. A book and a box illustrate how alternative pathways to mainstream medicine (in both childbirth and psychiatry) came to fruition in the 1970s.

A BOOK

In 1967, Joanne Santana, a self-proclaimed hippie living in San Jose, California, discovered she was pregnant at the age of twenty-one. "I really knew nothing about having a baby," she reflected later. Her only point of reference came from the popular television series *Wagon Train*. The Western featured a wagon train on its adventures from Missouri to California, focusing almost entirely on the masculine pursuits of the predominantly male cast. Every so often, however, as Santana recalls, "the wagons would pull over, you'd hear a woman scream, a baby cry, and the wagons would roll on. So I thought you screamed, and the baby came out. That was my childbirth education."[1]

Needless to say, the show did little to prepare her for her first birth, which took place in O'Connor Hospital, the oldest hospital in Santa Clara County. It was a quick labor. Santana was already seven centimeters dilated by the time she checked in, and a labor nurse assured her she would make it to the requisite ten centimeters soon enough. But Santana found the pain to be nearly unendurable and begged for medication. "I thought the whole purpose of going to the hospital was that they give you something for pain," she remarked later. Instead, the nurse encouraged her to think about her breathing, which helped temporarily. Suddenly she felt she couldn't take the pain anymore, and the contractions stopped, triggering self-reflection. "And I'm sitting there going, well, what are my options here? And I thought well somehow my body has gotten pregnant, grown this child, well on the way to having this baby, and I did not understand intellectually how to do this, but my body evidently is doing it, so I've gotta trust my body that it's going to get me out of this." The contractions began again and she felt the urge to push. Because the doctor had not yet arrived, the nurse instructed her not to push. Hospital staff wheeled her into a delivery room and strapped down her arms and legs. As Santana remembered it, this happened right after she had made a deal with herself to listen to her body. "So this is not good, but I'm trying to be a good girl trying not to push and stuff. And when [the doctor] finally gets there he cuts a huge mediolateral episiotomy for a six-pound, fourteen ounce little girl I should have had fifteen minutes ago with the nurses. I could not sit down for a month without a pillow."[2] She left with her new healthy baby girl, Jordana, feeling dazed by her birth experience and anything but empowered.

A year later, Santana picked up the underground newspaper *San Francisco Express Times* and learned about a class taught by Stephen Gaskin offered through the experimental college at San Francisco State. "Monday

Night Class" was a series of lectures covering everything from meditation to discussions about politics, religion, and psychedelics. "When we first got the class together we were like a research instrument, and we read everything we could on religion, magic, superstition, ecology, extrasensory perception, fairy tales, collective unconscious, folkways, and math and physics," Gaskin recalled. "And we began finding things out as we went along about the nature of the mind."[3] By 1969, this class had grown to several thousand people, many of whom began to see Gaskin as their spiritual teacher.

At first glance, Stephen Gaskin does not appear to be hippie guru material. Born in 1935, he served in the Marine Corps in Korea as a rifleman in the early 1950s. He moved to San Francisco where he attended San Francisco State College under the G.I. bill, getting his B.A. in 1962 and M.A. in creative writing in 1964, then taught creative writing and semantics at the college until 1966 when his contract ran out. "It wasn't that I got fired for being a hippy," Gaskin explains, "it was just that I'd gotten too weird to rehire by the time my contract expired."[4] He approached the head of San Francisco State's Experimental College and found out that there was a teaching slot available on Monday nights. "The idea was to compare notes with other trippers about tripping and the whole psychic and psychedelic world," Gaskin, by then heavily caught up in the San Francisco countercultural scene, writes. "We discussed love, sex, dope, God, gods, war, peace, enlightenment, mindcop, free will and what-have-you, all in a stoned, truthful, hippie atmosphere. We studied religions, fairy tales, legends, children's stories, the I Ching, Zen koans—and tripping." Everything was fair game in his multidisciplinary approach—including, and especially, psychedelics.

Psychiatric research on LSD and other psychoactive substances had been on the increase over the past decade, as studies suggested their therapeutic potential.[5] Gaskin and his Monday Night followers also believed in the therapeutic potential of psychedelics, but in a different context. According to Gaskin, psychedelics served as a catalyst to expand human consciousness and attain greater spiritual awareness. Thus, drugs (initially LSD, but then natural substances peyote and psilocybin) were a regular part of Monday Night class, as well as Sunday Morning Services (standing meditations) held before sunrise in Sutro Park. According to one follower, "Sunday Service was considered an ideal place to trip—a peaceful oasis in time, where the energy was dependably high, the vibes good, and of course, there was Stephen—tripping guide extraordinaire."[6]

Joanne Santana became a regular attendant in 1969. When she found she was pregnant later that year, she sought recommendations from other attendees regarding alternative birth practitioners, determined to have a different experience the second time around. Santana learned that there was a man named Bob who was calling himself a midwife living at the Good Earth commune on Pine Street in the Haight-Ashbury district. Six weeks before her due date, on Mother's Day of 1970, she went to meet him. "It was quite a scene," she recalled.[7] By this time, Haight-Ashbury had been overrun by heroin and speed junkies, and many of the Haight's founding hippies had moved on. Founded in 1968 by two ex-convicts, the Good Earth was part of the second wave of the Haight's hippie settlements. With membership ever changing, over seven hundred people flowed through the commune's half-dozen houses in the neighborhood.[8] In honor of Mother's Day, the men were baking bread and the women were "taking long baths and lounging around," which was an exception in the largely male-dominant counterculture movement.[9] It was perhaps fitting that the "midwife" Santana went to meet was male, since that, too, was nearly unheard of.

Bob had long stringy gray hair and looked to be in his forties. He asked Santana about her previous birth experience and assured her she could give birth without an episiotomy this time around. In the forty-odd deliveries Bob had presided over, he had never done an episiotomy, recommending instead a slow delivery and an ice pack to prevent tearing. Unfortunately, Bob was about to move to a commune in Oregon and could not assist with Santana's birth, but he sent her to the New Age Foods store to purchase a midwifery manual he found useful.

Fred Rohe, originally a chemicals salesman, had opened New Age Foods back in 1965 in Haight Ashbury. A self-declared Buddhist interested in "providing nutritional and spiritual guidance," he offered everything from herbal tea to books, record albums, and a meditation area. By 1969, his sales had increased tenfold, indicative of the growing marketability of countercultural items.[10] On the shelf of his store sat a small book, *Pregnancy, Childbirth, and the Newborn: A Manual for Rural Midwives,* written by a Stanford thoracic surgeon, Dr. Leo Eloesser.

Santana leafed through the manual before taking it home. "It was just our speed," she later recalled. "It's like 'put warm brick in baby's bed. Remove brick before putting baby in bed.' It told you how to do you know a birthing pack, how to sterilize your instruments, how to deliver a breech birth, how to stop a hemorrhage, things like that."[11] Santana did not realize it at the time of her purchase, but this little manual would become crucial to her and her community of Gaskin followers.

How did a manual for rural midwives end up in an urban natural foods store? The book began as a series of teaching papers used in midwifery training courses in communist-controlled areas of northern China, where doctors were in extremely short supply. The context could not have been more different. While Santana sought to escape from the clutches of modern obstetrics, Dr. Leo Eloesser, residing less than sixteen miles away and teaching at one of the country's most prestigious medical schools,

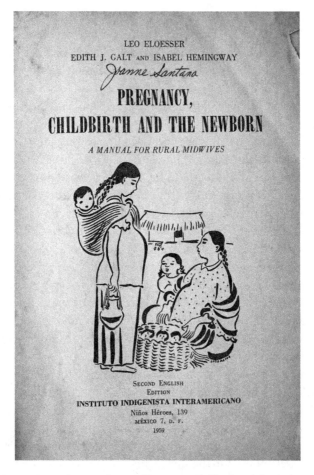

Figure 3.1 Joanne Santana's personal copy of *Pregnancy, Childbirth, and the Newborn*. Photograph by Wendy Kline.

carried his expertise to war-torn rural north China in an effort to improve infant and maternal mortality rates. According to Eloesser, in 1948 there was one doctor for every 80,000 to 150,000 inhabitants, resulting in dire conditions.[12] As part of a UNICEF mission, Eloesser agreed to create a medical training program in northern China to improve the situation.[13]

Eloesser faced an enormous task. The $500,000 allocated for this mission could not produce the kind of facilities or personnel available in the West. Approximately fifty medical schools generated somewhere between one and two hundred "acceptably trained" and a thousand "ill-trained" graduates per year, and at that rate, Eloesser argued, "graduates would die off faster than they could be replaced."[14] Some alternative body of health workers needed to fill that gap. He proposed the creation of a new medical program in north China involving the recruitment of young men and women with no more than a grade school education. Six-month training courses in sanitation, communicable diseases, and midwifery would produce competent health care practitioners in a practical and efficient manner. Three months of "simple" classwork followed by supervised field work in each of these areas, he claimed, would dramatically improve health outcomes.[15] As UNICEF was quick to point out in a later press release touting the program's success, it "reversed the usual procedure of selecting only a few for top-level training, frequently given outside of their country."[16] After training, these "average level" students would in turn train others in nearby villages, thereby spreading basic training models further out into the countryside. While this process would become common after Mao's 1965 directive for the widespread establishment of "barefoot doctors" in China's rural areas, the medical training program created by Eloesser seventeen years earlier set a clear precedent.[17]

But how would he go about teaching these new courses? Eloesser himself had no background in midwifery, nor was he likely to be exposed to it in the United States. Ironically, the increasing embrace of Western medicine in the early twentieth century led to the rapid growth in the professionalization of midwifery in China, but not in the United States. Rural midwives in China had neither the resources nor the access to the Western-funded modern training centers such as the Central Midwifery Schools in Nanjing or Beijing.[18] Like the aging African-American midwives in the rural American South, these rural Chinese midwives were referred to by public health officials as "Granny Midwives" and were frequently perceived as part of the public health problem rather than part of the solution.[19] Instead, Eloesser sought the "hitherto untapped reservoir of woman power" of the student population to practice what he called "sensible midwifery." They could, for example, "sit by at a normal delivery and refrain from putting cow dung or earth on a newborn's navel," a derogatory reference to the practices of local midwives that he deemed backward and unsanitary.[20]

For teachers, Eloesser contacted the American Board Mission in Tientsin, a Christian missionary organization that had established several centers in northern China by the late nineteenth century. This particular mission had two nurse midwives, Isabel Hemingway and Edith Galt, who were available to come teach for Eloesser. Both Hemingway and Galt had grown up in China with missionary parents, spoke the language fluently, and studied nursing and midwifery at the Maternity Center in New York City where they had "obstetrical training in modern New York hospitals."[21] They thus represented in Eloesser's view the best of both worlds—training in Western medicine and experience with the local culture.

Eloesser, Hemingway, and Galt put together a series of teaching papers to present to their Chinese students, who numbered twenty young women in 1949 and another nineteen in 1950. The basic text was accompanied by sixty-six illustrations and covered anatomy, fetal development, labor and delivery, postpartum care, and hygiene. Isabel Hemingway later commented privately to Eloesser on how effective this teaching style had been. "I know that students learned the steps for delivery and did the things they would have to do several times in class so that when they really saw a delivery they were already knowing what to expect. It was a great help to them and to us."[22]

Eloesser's UNICEF mission proved short-lived; he supervised only two series of medical training courses lasting just over a year. Galt moved on to Korea, Hemingway to Turkey, and Eloesser to Mexico. Their dispersion helped to further disseminate the principles of the manual, which continued to be revised, expanded, and translated over the next twenty-six years. Evidence suggests that the book's impact was felt not just in developing countries, but also in the United States. "In regard to your manual for rural midwives, I purchased quite a number of these when they came out and have distributed quite a few," noted Dr. Nicholas Eastman, chief of obstetrics at Johns Hopkins University Hospital in 1956.[23] Nearly two decades later, Dr. Victor Richards of San Francisco Children's Hospital also expressed his enthusiasm to Eloesser. "You would be surprised, but I have heard over the years many favorable comments about your manual for rural midwives. I am delighted to know you will be putting out a new edition."[24]

Taught in China by American missionaries, published in Spanish, English, Korean, and Portuguese, this manual reached a global market, but also landed in a health food store just a few miles away from its creator's home institution. By the mid-1970s, it was commonly used at the Santa Cruz Birth Center by young activist midwives.[25] More than a decade before the first edition of *Our Bodies, Ourselves* would offer lay readers an accessible manual on women's health and trigger a women's health movement, *Pregnancy, Childbirth, and the Newborn* became a do-it-yourself tool that provided the necessary foundation for a burgeoning home birth movement. Yet unlike the women's health activists who wrote *Our Bodies, Ourselves* in the 1970s, Dr. Leo Eloesser had no intention of providing urban hippies with an alternative to modern obstetrical care.

Armed with her new manual, Santana continued her search for a birth attendant. Another Gaskin follower told her about a labor and delivery nurse, Diane Mehler, who later became considered "the Monday Night Class midwife" and had recently delivered a baby at home.[26] "And so I went to see her," Santana recalled. Mehler lived in a house near the top of Mount Tamalpais (along with the psychedelic rock band Sopwith Camel), about twenty-five miles north of San Francisco. Newly pregnant herself, Mehler agreed to help the couple, but explained that she did not want to have to do it in San Jose because of the long drive and Santana's short first labor. So the couple moved into an old schoolbus to allow for greater portability. On July 4, 1970, two weeks after her due date, Santana and her family were headed to Sutro Park to hear Gaskin speak when she had several strong contractions. They turned the bus around and headed to a friend's house in San Francisco to call Diane. When they couldn't reach her, they called the Good Earth commune and spoke to a woman whose baby had been delivered by Bob, and she agreed to come over and help. Upon her arrival, she filled the tub with warm water and helped Santana climb in. "The water was great," Santana recalled. They finally reached Diane, who came over, boiled her instruments, and helped Santana out of the tub to check on her progress. Baby Anthony was already on his way out, born in only three hours. In the distance, Independence Day fireworks seemed to announce Anthony's arrival. In exchange for Diane's services, Santana gave her their 52-inch round Mexican oak kitchen table and baby cradle.

Santana remembers her birthing experience as a major turning point in her life. "It was the most empowering thing that ever happened to me," she explained. "The difference between those two births was just night and day," she said of Jordana and Anthony's births. "I just felt kind of ripped off after Jordana. I mean it was wonderful having her, and she was a great nurser and all that stuff but I didn't feel like empowered where they took her away right away. I wasn't allowed to have her to just nurse her when I wanted, I'd get engorged, and I'd have to wait for them to bring her." Her recovery time with Anthony's birth was dramatically shorter. "This time I could sit right up, no stitches, you know, it was just incredible. And I felt like a monkey, I felt like I could do anything." More significantly, she found her calling. "I really wanted to devote my life to bringing that empowerment to families. Because I don't care if people want to have 'em in the hospital or a birth center or at home but I think it should be their choice."[27] Santana was one of a growing number of women in the counterculture whose own birth experiences helped to revive the practice of midwifery in the United States.

The following Sunday, Santana and her family made it to Sutro Park for Stephen Gaskin's regular Sunday service. Sitting in the shade of a palm tree was thirty-year-old Ina May Middleton (who would later marry Stephen Gaskin). Santana proudly presented her friend with newborn Anthony. When Ina May asked where she had had the baby, Santana told her that she did it at home. "And she said well how did you do that and I said with a midwife. And you could just see her eyes light up and the wheels start turning and she said 'oh it would be really nice to have one of those, you know.'"[28]

Like 99 percent of all American mothers in the 1960s, Ina May's first birth experience had taken place in a hospital. "Fear of having a repeat of what I experienced during my first birth in a hospital was what prompted me to figure out a way to learn to be a midwife," she later declared.[29] While attending graduate school in Illinois, she had delivered her daughter in a hospital, an experience that traumatized her. "During birth at the hospital, I was left alone and treated like I had done something nasty. Then I was approached by a gang of masked attendants who came in the room and treated me like a ritual victim. They used forceps, and then I wasn't allowed to see my baby for 18 hours," she remembers.[30]

Ina May was raised in Marshalltown, Iowa, and after receiving her Bachelor's degree from the University of Iowa, she traveled to Malaysia with her first husband (whom she married at the age of nineteen) to volunteer for the Peace Corps. They planned to head directly to San Francisco after two years in Malaysia, but when they discovered she was pregnant, they decided to return to the Midwest. "We thought, well, you don't just go out pregnant and decide to become a hippie with no way to make a living." With a master's degree, she could work as a teaching assistant for better pay. After obtaining a degree in English from Northern Illinois University in 1967, she took off with her husband and young daughter for San Francisco to "become hippies," as she remembered later.[31]

She found work in Chinatown, teaching English to local residents, while her husband stayed home with their daughter. "I absolutely loved that job," she recalled.[32] Like so many who flocked to San Francisco in the 1960s, her world was soon turned upside down. She and her husband began attending Stephen Gaskin's Monday Night Class, where she first encountered the man who would become her mentor and eventually her life partner. She also met her future midwifery partner Pamela Hunt, an art major at San Francisco State who had taken one of Gaskin's very first courses, "Magic, Einstein, and God," in 1966. Hunt recalls that there were only eight or nine people in the class, though within a few years that figure would grow to 1,500. "We talked about telepathy and how people interact with each other on a vibrational level as well as a physical level and how important it was to take care of the energy that you are dealing with," she remembers. These ideas would prove to be enormously beneficial a few years later as she began to apply them to coping with contractions in labor.

Though Hunt had not yet given birth, her exposure to hospital birth practices, like Santana and Ina May, had a profound effect on the path she chose to take. As an art major, she studied at the University of Guadalajara for two years in the early 1960s, where she took a required anatomy course. On a field trip to a state-run hospital, Hunt witnessed three births. "When they delivered the babies, they kind of pulled the babies out, tossed them up in the air, slapped them on the back a couple of times and threw them to a nurse," she recalled.[33] Each of the mothers looked "tired and forlorn" afterwards, with no one to comfort them, as husbands weren't allowed in the room. Yet there was Pamela, along with her classmates, "a group of strangers who didn't know the first thing about birth," witnessing the entire event. "Why they arranged for us to be at these births and put these poor women up as models at this most vulnerable time in their lives, I'll never know. We certainly didn't learn any anatomy, or compassion for the mother or baby, either."[34] She discovered that the cesarean section rate in Mexico was 75 percent, which she found shocking, as she "expected Mexico to be pretty natural."[35]

Hunt returned to her hometown of Sacramento after two years in Mexico, intending to complete her undergraduate degree at California State University Sacramento. But in 1966, she "got mixed up with a guy" that her mother did not like and headed down to San Francisco to finish her coursework there. "When I first got to San Francisco I was as square as they come. And all of a sudden I was in the middle of the art department at San Francisco State in 1966. And that changed everything." She signed up for Stephen Gaskin's class that included meditation and discussions about politics, religion, and psychedelics. "The world changed overnight," she says. "Literally."[36]

"OUT TO SAVE THE WORLD": THE CARAVAN

In 1970, while preaching at the nondenominational Glide Church, Stephen Gaskin was invited to deliver a series of lectures at schools and churches across the country. More than 200 of his followers decided to join him in school buses for this "Astral Continental Congress," a call for a spiritual and social revolution. The Caravan, as it came to be called, generated more and more media attention as its collection of school buses wound their way through forty-two states spreading the inchoate messages of peace and spiritual and social revolution to students and churchgoers. Remarkably, despite his sometimes rambling messages and sermons, Gaskin provided a logic and rationale for his vision of peace based on both spirituality and science.

At the age of thirty-five, Gaskin was older than many of his followers, yet his style and strategy attracted countercultural youth. "Stephen said things I had always known but had never heard anyone articulate before," remembers Cara Gillette. "He talked about energy, God, attention, and compassion. I felt, inside my mind, a clear bell of truth."[37] He spoke in plain language, mixing modern-day metaphors of science and spirituality in his attempts to provide simple answers to complex questions. "Religion is the wiring diagram of the way human energy is moved to relate with the universe," he explained on Halloween of 1970 at St. Stephen's Catholic Church in Minneapolis.[38] In Iowa City, he described the human soul as "the electrical field that surrounds your equipment," while the "brain is a field generator, it's not just a hunk of meat with wiring in it."[39] Speaking at the Washington Monument, he reflected, "I was thinking this morning that praying is like communicating telepathically."[40] Natural hallucinogens such as peyote or psylocibin enabled Gaskin and his followers to experience enhanced awareness and appreciation for connections between mind, body, and spirit.[41]

Intent on showing the media and the mainstream that hippies were anything but lazy or stupid, Gaskin demonstrated their potential for complexity by blurring the boundaries between religion, spirituality, and science. Yet the heart of his message was quite simple and practical (if only loosely based on specific scientific principles). "Spiritual isn't like misty or somewhere else. Spiritual is how do we, here and now, work it out as best as we can, because this is all we have," he explained to students at Wright State University in Dayton, Ohio on November 16.[42] Speaking primarily to youth upset by the Vietnam War and social injustices at home, Gaskin urged them to do something. "I feel like beatniks have been spaced long enough, and that we know where it's at, and that it's time we got off welfare, gave up food stamps, and began to produce with this energy which we say we have so much of."[43]

Well aware of the media attention he was getting on the Caravan, he took the opportunity to portray the counterculture as full of positive potential for social change. Just before dawn on December 27, Gaskin maneuvered the fifty-odd buses of the Caravan through the streets of Washington D.C. to the Ellipse, the park between the White House and the Washington Monument, for a sunrise service. One Caravan member reflected that their arrival was "one of those moments, full of meaning and symbolism, pregnant with possibilities."[44] CBS news was on hand to interview Gaskin, and the *Washington Post* covered the story as well.

At a time when many mainstream Americans associated hippiedom with hedonism, Gaskin and his followers sought to convey a much more activist mindset. As if to remind onlookers that Gaskin was doing much more than "tuning in and dropping out," the destination sign on top of his Scenicruiser read "Out to Save the World." This group believed that they carried an inclusive message relevant to everyone—male or female, rich or poor, black or white. One member, Michael Traugot, described the sense of optimism and importance that these travelers experienced as they crossed the country:

Several times on the Caravan Stephen had told us that we were living at a very unique time, a crossroads, an unusual moment in history. So much change was happening, people felt so confused and so desperate, so hungry for understanding, that a window was temporarily opened into their hearts and minds. People would listen to new ideas, consider points of view they would not have considered before. We had a chance to influence our culture, the group mind of America and the world, in the direction of peace and compassion and living with nature rather than trying to dominate. That's why we were doing this Caravan. But we had better act quickly, Stephen would tell us, because the window might soon close, the culture harden up again.

And it was working! Everywhere we went, the authorities and the mainstream society as a whole were very sweet to us, treated us with a great deal of respect. We had the highest spiritual and ethical standards, went out of our way to be and appear harmless, to show respect to others, to work hard and not ask for handouts. All this worked in our favor, but it wasn't just us. It was partly the times.[45]

The excitement was palpable, and the potential for change seemed enormous. People were listening, and they appeared willing to consider what Gaskin had to say as a legitimate alternative to the status quo (participating in psychedelic experiences undoubtedly enhanced their receptivity). What they did not realize at the time, however, is that the longest lasting impact of the Caravan had less to do with Stephen than it did with some of his pregnant female followers, whose determination to stay out of the hospital led to a revolution in birth practices. When Gaskin announced his plan to speak across the country, follower Cara Gillette was pregnant. "I knew I had to go with Stephen and the community," she remembers. "The thought of staying behind and having my baby in some hospital, with 'sharp things coming at me', wasn't an option for me. I wasn't so much scared of having a baby as of those 'sharp things coming at me'."[46] Her birth story would become memorialized in The Farm's publication *Spiritual Midwifery*, introducing hundreds of thousands of readers to the idea that medical doctors were not the only ones capable of delivering babies in modern America.

BIRTHS ON THE CARAVAN

Just like in the *Wagon Train* television series of Joanne Santana's childhood, when a woman went into labor, the Caravan pulled over, waited for the birth, then rolled on. "We all parked in a sort of protective formation around the bus in which the birth would take place," wrote Gaskin, "and everyone waited for the baby's first cry."[47] The first baby was born in a parking lot at Northwestern University, while Gaskin was lecturing to several hundred people in an auditorium. Franz, the father, approached Gaskin to ask for his assistance during the labor (because he had received first aid training in Korea), but since he was scheduled to lecture, Ina May offered to help instead. "I was no midwife at the time," she wrote later, "but I was able to help the mother [Anna] stay relaxed." She brought fellow Caravanners Pamela Hunt, Mary Louise Perkins, and Margaret Nofziger with her to help in the small bus, lit by kerosene lamps. "I remember her looking beautiful all through her labor," remembered Pamela, "kind of rosy and glowing."[48] The labor only lasted three hours, and baby Immanuel came out without any problems, caught by his father.

After the birth, Ina May felt stunned. "I was in a state of amazement for several days," she wrote later. "I had never seen a newborn baby before (my baby was almost a day old before I was allowed to see her) and I was struck with how perfect this baby looked. . . . I felt a definite calling to be a midwife, but my master's degree in English had not prepared me for anything so real life as a birth."[49] In order to gain a better sense of the mechanics of birth, she turned to the resource available to her on the Caravan—Eloesser's *Pregnancy, Childbirth and the Newborn.*

Cara Gillette felt lucky to witness this first Caravan birth, knowing that she, too, would give birth on the road. "Anna was so lovely," she remembers of the laboring mother.[50] What she did not expect was to be next in line, as her due date was six weeks away when she felt some cramps the following week. The Caravan was stopped at Bruin Lakes State Park outside of Ann Arbor, Michigan. "We were concerned because it was so early," Cara explained, "and we didn't want to admit that it was really happening."[51] She scrambled to prepare for the birth. She had scraped together her and her partner Michael's small savings to buy a tiny bread truck to travel in the Caravan, and it had broken down several times on the trip. "We were constantly falling behind," she remembers.[52] It was too small for a birth, so Mary Louise Perkins, who had also been at the first Caravan birth, and her partner Joseph lent them their bus for the day.

As soon as she lay down in Perkins's bed, twenty-five people crowded onto the bus to witness the second Caravan birth. One of the men even had a camera. Pamela Hunt recalled that the "vibes felt strained."[53] Sensing Cara's discomfort, she and Ina May asked all of the men to leave except Michael, the father of Cara's child. Though Cara's twin sister Mary had been traveling on the Caravan with her husband, they were stuck in Minneapolis rebuilding the engine of their van.[54] Pamela and Ina May hunkered down with the manual to prepare for the impending birth, keenly aware that it would be a premature one. Then suddenly, one of the other women there "became nervous and superstitious when she saw what I was reading, and took the book out my hands," Ina May recalled, "afraid that if I read about something negative, I would cause it to happen." What happened next taught her the importance of accepting responsibility. "Instead of taking the book back, I allowed myself to be intimidated by the other woman." [55] According to Hunt, "the situation felt shaky."[56]

Yet Cara Gillette labored along, finding the birthing to be "surprisingly easy . . . It felt ecstatic. Everything that happened in my body felt really natural."[57] Shortly before baby Anne was born, she began to doubt herself. "I wasn't sure I could do it." Then one woman took her hand, and another massaged her feet. "The loving touch made all the difference," Cara remembers. "I pushed through."[58] Baby Anne was born after six hours of labor, weighing just five pounds, and caught by her father. She promptly "gave a small cry and then turned blue and just lay there."[59] Panic ensued. The women had not yet read what to do if the baby didn't breathe. "We all watched, frozen," recalls Cara.[60] Someone ran out and got Stephen, who rushed over and breathed into the baby's mouth. "She took a breath, cried, and turned pink; our first miracle and our first heavy lesson," recalled Hunt.[61] Gillette, eternally grateful to Stephen, reflected, "it was probably a good thing we learned the high stakes of birth early on."[62] Perhaps this scare had an impact on their own midwifery manual; they listed terms that pertained to birthing emergencies in easy-to-find bold print in the index of *Spiritual Midwifery*.

By the third birth, which took place in Ripley, New York, Ina May was officially established as the midwife in charge, and the only people allowed to be present for a birth were the female attendants (Ina May, Pamela, and Margaret) and the father of the child. This time, the Caravan pulled over on the side of the road in the middle of the town to await the baby's birth, close to a church. After Ina May delivered the baby, the minister rang the church bells, and the locals greeted the new mother with food and warm wishes, a reminder that the alternative practices espoused by these itinerant hippies were not always met with hostility.

Eight more births would take place during the Caravan, each one generating excitement described by Ina May as "contagious." Pamela and Ina May were among the pregnant women who learned from those before them. "Each mother who gave birth became an inspiring and encouraging example to the other women," wrote Ina May. "We came to look at birth as a sort of initiation or rite of passage—something for which you could gather up your courage with the help of your friends and contemporaries."[63]

But in order for birth to become a truly inspirational event, it had to be safe. Beginning with the premature Ann Arbor birth, Ina May realized that for all of the beauty and naturalness of birth, it sometimes required medical expertise. Santana's midwifery manual was a start, but the group lacked anyone with hands-on training until the Caravan reached Rhode

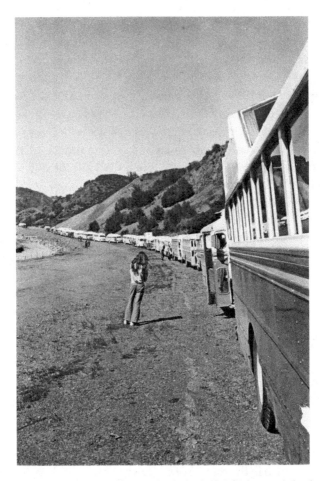

Figure 3.2 The Caravan on April 1, 1971, just after the birth of Phil Schweitzer's daughter Sara Jean. Photograph by Gerald Wheeler. Reprinted by permission.

Island. There, a local obstetrician named Louis La Pere, who had read about the Caravan and the births en route, came to visit and offered Ina May, Hunt, and Nofziger a hands-on seminar on birthing emergencies and complications. La Pere had studied medicine at the University of Bologna in the early 1950s before returning to his home town of Westerly, Rhode Island.[64] Perhaps his interest in Ina May's endeavors was a result of his European education and the fact that the University of Bologna had long had an established midwifery program. Whatever the case, he taught the three aspiring midwives sterile technique, how to resuscitate a newborn, and what to do with an umbilical cord that became tightly wrapped around the baby's neck. He also gave them obstetrical instruments, medications, and an obstetrics textbook. "It was a little handbook," she recalled. "Benson's

Handbook of Obstetrics and Gynecology." She shared the book with Pamela, who would read it for a couple of weeks and then pass it back to Ina May to study it.[65] "And so I used it kind of as a guide," Gaskin explained, viewing La Pere as one of "a bunch of doctors that really thought that the U.S. had missed the boat in not having midwives. And thought that that was going to change."[66] Like the residents of Ripley, New York, Dr. La Pere seemed to view births on the buses as a potentially revolutionary act deserving of recognition.

Thus, like Stephen Gaskin, Ina May viewed her new calling as a mixture of science, practicality, and spirituality. Her approach to birth reflected his philosophy. This is of course not surprising, given their relationship. Not only were they partners (they would officially marry in 1976), they were also a team, and in the spring of 1974, Stephen ordained Ina May as "acting minister" to be able to conduct services in his absence.[67] In her view, birth was "telepathic," "heavy," and a "trip." One's mindset and relationship with the universe affected the birth process, as it did all aspects of life. "Putting out energy from one end of your tube (in the form of truth or love)," she explained, "makes it easy to put out energy from the other end (in the form of a baby). The reverse of this is true too—if a lady squinches up her mouth so that it isn't good to look at or screams or says pissed off things, her puss will cinch up too, and she'll be more likely to tear." Quoting the founder of the Sufi movement in the West, she added, " 'with love, even the rocks will open.'"[68] Thus, spirituality also had a practical element, according to Gaskin, actually easing some of the pain of childbirth. Childbirth, in turn, provided a spiritual, potentially transformational, experience for the mother. This revelation would prove essential not only for the rebirth of midwifery in America, but also for the rise of an entirely different profession: transpersonal psychology, under the leadership of Czech psychiatrist Stan Grof.

THE FARM

At the end of the tour, Gaskin and his followers decided to purchase land in Tennessee and create a commune on a thousand acres, based on his principles. They were only back in San Francisco for a week before they turned around and headed back east, becoming "Okies in reverse."[69] The sense of community that had been developed along the route turned into something more permanent as they plowed, farmed, built, and meditated together. As scholar Fred Turner points out, this was in the midst of the "largest wave of communalization in American history." Perhaps as many as 750,000 Americans lived in some ten thousand communes in the early 1970s, though few survived as long as The Farm. Turner refers to these pioneer

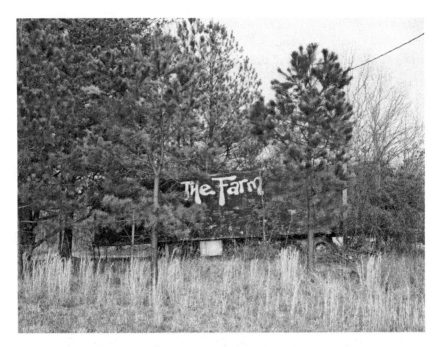

Figure 3.3 The Farm in 2013. Photograph by Wendy Kline.

visionaries as "New Communalists," arguing that even as they opted to live apart from mainstream society, they often "embraced the collaborative social practices, the celebration of technology, and the cybernetic rhetoric of mainstream military-industrial-academic research."[70] This is certainly true of The Farm, where ingenuity, creativity, and determination led to a great deal of innovation: the first hand-held Geiger counter (called the "Nuke Buster"), rechargeable electric golf carts, and even a Doppler fetal pulse detector.[71] As Farm resident Phil Schweitzer recalls, "the interest in all of this stuff to me is the fact that we did it on no budget. Not that the technology didn't exist—we were just trying to use the scraps from society to piece together the technology that we would need to survive out here in the woods with no money."[72]

With more babies on the way, one of the first orders of business was to establish a protocol for deliveries on The Farm. One thousand acres was a lot of space, and after living in such tight quarters for the previous four months, many families scattered to the far ends of the property. Initially, this proved challenging to Ina May and Hunt, who "had no communications other than how loud we could shout from hill to hill to relay a message. If we needed to make a phone call, we had to drive out three miles to a local bar to use the phone."[73] Once phone lines were established, midwives and pregnant women received priority in getting a line installed. Later, each midwife was provided with a pickup truck or four-wheel-drive vehicle equipped with a citizen's band radio so that they could be in constant communication. "We were always very techie," Hunt remembers.[74]

Shortly after they settled on The Farm, a public health nurse visited the premises. Eager to maintain their practice of delivering babies, Ina May asked her how they could receive more training to practice midwifery in Tennessee. Though plenty of home births occurred in the region, as a large Amish community lived nearby, Tennessee had no licensure program for midwives. The nurse returned the following day with two men from the Bureau of Vital Statistics. "She gave me a box of ampules of silver nitrate [to drop in the newborns' eyes], and the men gave me a stack of birth certificates and death certificates and wished me good luck." This goodwill gesture gave them a boost of confidence that they could continue with their craft. It also made them realize that they had not obtained birth certificates for all of the babies born on the Caravan, a task that proved challenging, since many public health authorities "weren't sure how to go about certifying the birth of a baby who had arrived in a schoolbus." [75] Most newborns had been weighed on produce scales in nearby grocery stores, hardly an official indicator of a child's heft.

Since midwifery school was not an option, Ina May and the "midwife crew" turned to the local family practitioner, Dr. John Williams. While relations between doctors and lay midwives in the 1970s were frequently hostile, that was not the case between Williams and The Farm midwives. Shortly after they arrived, the midwives brought one of their newborns who had been born prematurely to Dr. Williams. "He took a liking to us," Pamela remembers, "and so he started coming out here." She describes him as "a real doctor," referring to his warmth, caring, and concern. "And he was not afraid to teach us."[76] In addition to practicing at Maury Regional Hospital, Williams had been delivering babies in the homes of local Amish families for years and had noticed that the Amish women and their babies carried a lower rate of infection than those he delivered in the hospital. He theorized that home birth mothers had built up resistance to organisms in their own home that made them less susceptible to infection, and he was eager to see "if his theory would be borne out by the statistics of [The Farm] births. (It was.)," declared Ina May. "We were told to call him any time, night or day, if we had questions about the pregnant or birthing women and their babies."[77] Perhaps due to the rural setting and the lack of health care providers, country doctors were more likely to view midwives with any level of experience as helpmeets rather than hindrances, allowing for a more collaborative approach to birth.

Thus began a decades-long fruitful relationship between Dr. Williams and The Farm midwives, who consulted with him regularly on everything

from fevers to breech births. "Dr. Williams helped us a lot," recalled Hunt.
"He always made you feel good." When he got a CB radio for his pickup
truck so that they could reach him when he was away from a telephone, his
radio nickname was "Dr. Feelgood."[78] His reputation extended beyond the
boundaries of The Farm; in 1981, he was selected by *Good Housekeeping
Magazine* as one of the nation's Ten Most Outstanding Family Physicians.[79]
"He was an inspiration to many people in our community and to me," wrote
former patient Debbie O'Neal. "I have many fond memories of him. I remember how he always cared for my grandparents and my parents. I do not
know of another doctor that had as much care and concern for others as he
did."[80] He himself was modest about what he had done for the community
of midwives, writing to Ina May toward the end of his career, "Any help
I gave to you was a part of every physician's creed—i.e., to learn, to experience, then to teach—too many of us forget."[81]

With his assistance, in the first two years the midwife crew established
their prenatal clinic, using equipment donated by doctors, along with some
purchased at a nearby medical supply house; delivered 129 babies; and continued their studies. "All this time we were reading obstetrics textbooks and
learning everything we could about the technical part," Ina May wrote. "We
learned more about the vibes part with every birthing that we attended."[82]

The crew itself changed over the years, and some women rotated in and
out of midwifery positions, either to care for their children or do other
types of work on The Farm. Joanne Santana was originally a teacher at The
Farm school, transitioning over to the midwife crew as her children grew
older and more independent. The team consisted of much more than the
actual midwives—they also had assistants. "You know, you hear about the
people in the book and stuff but there was a lot of people on the crew that
did nothing except go to the births, set up equipment, pack sterile packs
at the clinic, help out the clinic ladies working the pharmacy, it was a huge
crew behind every one of these births. Work as EMTs, do the ambulance
shifts, that kind of thing."[83] Together, as they developed their unique style,
blending science and spirituality, they believed that their relationship with
the medical community became more reciprocal.

This was particularly true when laboring mothers ended up in the hospital, most typically for a premature or breech birth, which happened four
times in the first two years. In many parts of the country, hippies in labor
begun at home and dealing with emergences were greeted at hospitals with
hostility—blamed for being irresponsible for attempting a home birth. But
in Summertown, Tennessee, the unusual mixture of people made for strange
bedfellows, colorful stories, and, sometimes, greater acceptance. Shortly
after the Caravan arrived at The Farm, two babies, Naomi and Brian, were
born prematurely and needed to spend time in the hospital. While there,

they served as young cultural ambassadors, for it was through them that their parents and midwives interacted with the community at large. "We got to be friends with a lot of Tennesseeans who we met while visiting the babies in the hospital," stated Ina May. "The nurses called Naomi 'the littlest hippy' and were fascinated that the babies had been born at home." These types of interactions potentially generated a greater understanding and appreciation for the two different perspectives on birth.

WRITING *SPIRITUAL MIDWIFERY*

As The Farm's population grew (up to 1,500 in 1982, with about 14,000 visitors per year), so did the number of births. Over 2,500 babies have been born on The Farm by the midwives, whose favorable statistics (including a 1.8 percent cesarean section rate) have caught the attention of consumers and birth practitioners around the world.[84] The Farm midwives also regularly offer workshops and training, such as a weeklong midwifery assistant workshop pictured in Figures 3.4 and 3.5.

Many more births have been affected by Ina May's home birthing philosophy than those born on The Farm, however. *Spiritual Midwifery,*

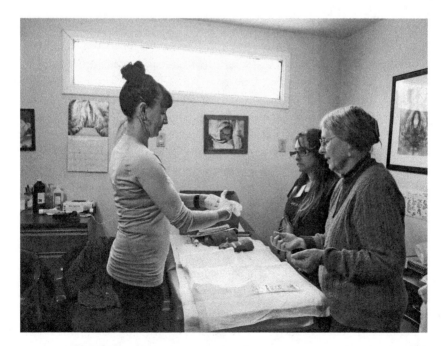

Figure 3.4 Pamela Hunt instructing two midwifery assistant students on sterile technique, March 25, 2013. Photograph by Wendy Kline. Reprinted by permission.

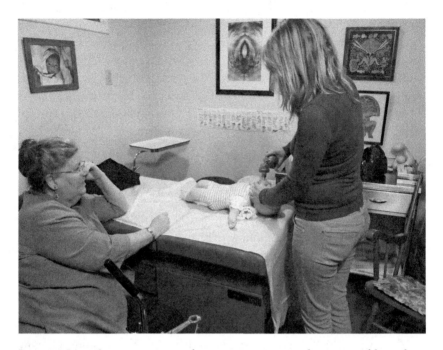

Figure 3.5 Joanne Santana instructing author on post-partum care and assessment of the newborn, March 29, 2013. Photograph by Siobhan Whalen.

a guide to birthing for consumers and birth practitioners published on The Farm, has sold over half a million copies, has been translated into six languages, and is still in print. *Spiritual Midwifery* started out as a section of The Book Publishing Company's first publication, *Hey Beatnik!* (1974). The earlier book provided an in-depth report about everything happening on The Farm, including its philosophy, farming, construction, soy dairy, grain mill, Farm Band, Motor Pool, school, and midwifery. This first version was only seventeen pages long (it would grow to 480 pages by the revised edition in 1977), a mixture of birth stories from multiple perspectives (father, mother, and midwife), photographs, instructions for prenatal care, and delivery.

It was not initially clear what form *Spiritual Midwifery* would take. Shortly after the publication of *Hey Beatnik!* Gaskin started receiving letters from readers asking for more information about home birth, along with more birth stories, and she realized she had material for an entire book. Looking at the birth stories written for *Hey Beatnik!,* she was struck by how good the writing was and decided to make these stories the centerpiece of *Spiritual Midwifery.* Hunt remembers, "we'd go out and pile on Ina May's bed and . . . we . . . started reading through the [birth stories] and you know I'd get to one and say 'oh this one's great—here, read this Ina

May' and . . . she'd read one and she'd start laughing and we'd all say 'yeah, we gotta put that one in.'"[85] Stories on breech births, hospital emergencies, and even stillbirths fleshed out the narrative, a sobering reminder of what could go wrong mixed in with the delight of a successful and empowering home birth.

Some of the letters Gaskin received made it clear that people were using her section in *Hey Beatnik!* to deliver their own babies. "And then I knew I had to write in a lot more detail." Thus, *Spiritual Midwifery* became much more than just a collection of birth stories for the expectant mother; it also served as a midwifery manual. Gaskin continued reading all that she could on the medical and technical aspects of birth, drawing on her newly established connections with nurses and doctors she had encountered both while traveling on the Caravan and on The Farm.[86] With this material, *Spiritual Midwifery* became a practical how-to manual and a spiritual guide. She divided it into three main sections: first, the birth stories (adding new ones in each edition); second, a section for the expectant parents (prenatal care, exercise, and taking care of a newborn); and finally, instructions to midwives (on anatomy and physiology, the stages of labor, complications, emergencies, and other important advice).[87]

PSYCHEDELIC BIRTH STORIES

In contrast to the standard descriptions of the agony of childbirth, birth stories published in *Spiritual Midwifery* were more likely to focus on the ecstasy. They also utilized the same hippie vocabulary used to describe drug experiences. "I laid down on the bed and began to rush and everything got psychedelic," described Mary of her labor on The Farm. "I began having beautiful, rushing contractions that started low, built up to a peak, and then left me floating about two feet off the bed." As her contractions intensified, they became more pleasurable. "It felt like I was making love to the rushes and I could wiggle my body and push into them and it was really fine." Whether or not Mary's experience accurately represented a typical birth on The Farm, it became the standard to aim for and was highlighted in the book as "a good description of how to handle the energy of the rushes of childbirth."[88] It was an intensely physical and emotional experience, thus inevitably heavily analyzed by Farm hippies as an opportunity for spiritual growth. Recall that Stephen Gaskin had been lecturing about the importance of energy back in 1966 in his "Magic, Einstein, and God" course at San Francisco State College, taken by midwife Pamela Hunt. The first midwives on The Farm were simply applying knowledge they had been exposed to for nearly a decade and that many had already experienced in a psychedelic state. With the right psychic tools, they believed, energy could be channeled into pleasure rather than pain.

Repeated references to psychedelic states during labor underscored the connections—whether literal or metaphorical—that Farm birthers perceived between the two. "I felt higher than I ever had in my life. It was such a heavy spiritual experience, and so much fun," wrote midwife Carol Nelson. "In between rushes I'd laugh at how telepathic it was."[89] In the proper setting, physical boundaries between the self/body and the external world could melt away. "I was somewhere on the astral plane, feeling all the forces of the Universe, it felt like, pounding my body," another wrote of her labor. "I flashed on wild stallions, thunder and lightning, and the ocean. I felt like my brain and upper body were separate from the rest of me, and were looking down on the action."[90]

Many stories featured in *Spiritual Midwifery* made references to communal out-of-body experiences that appeared to provide pain relief. "Mary Louise came over and put her attention totally to me. She and I swapped bodies," wrote Sheila. "It was far out. I felt myself leave and enter Mary Louise's and she came over and did a few contractions for me," she continued, believing that this process renewed her strength. It also transported her to another dimension. "I found myself in a beautiful place with a green field and a house. It was a place I'd never seen before. I could still tell my body was contracting, but I was detached from it. I told Mary Louise what happened and she said she'd been doing that contraction and had been able to feel it all."[91]

Recent studies point to evidence that validates out-of-body experiences (OBEs) as a "known and recognizable phenomenon" rather than illusory. Interestingly, current scholars attribute OBEs during childbirth as an indication of trauma, rather than as a coping mechanism or an expression of joy. Scholars perceive descriptions of women floating out of their bodies, observing the birth from above, as a form of dissociation or disembodiment, signifying current or past trauma.[92]

Clearly this was not what was being described in *Spiritual Midwifery*. In this context, birth was truly a communal experience—not just witnessed by others, but felt by others as well. This is part of what made it transformative. "We kept passing the energy between us, and Mary Louise knelt near my legs and Carol and Edward were on either side of me," wrote another woman in labor. "I'd rush and the energy would move up their spines and they'd arch their backs and straighten as they'd rush."[93] Birth, in this setting, provided a "contact high" for its participants that could guide them all toward greater spiritual awareness. "Maureen's birth was a very psychedelic experience for Joseph and me," wrote midwife Mary Louise. "She seemed to be filling us with her consciousness."[94] Birth provided, in the words of psychologist Abraham Maslow, a peak experience—those "powerful moments of clarity, joy, or religious ecstasy" that he wrote about in his influential 1964 volume, *Religions, Values, and Peak Experiences.*[95] Maslow described peak experiences as "rare, exciting, oceanic, deeply moving, exhilarating, elevating experiences that generate an advanced form of perceiving reality, and are even mystic and magical in their effect upon the experimenter."[96]

Psychedelic birth also strengthened the maternal–infant bond, according to its advocates. "I couldn't believe the strong bond I felt for my new baby and the overwhelming maternal instinct," wrote one new mother. She described the first moments with her newborn son as "paradise"; she was "mindblown" by his beauty and her love for him. Her description takes on a decidedly psychedelic tone. "The trees and the early morning light just flashed and reverbed like a strobe-light, and for several days I would have a flashback at every dawn and sunset. I was ecstatic for two weeks."[97]

Perhaps the most profound aspect of the birth experience described within the pages of *Spiritual Midwifery* was its ability to instill a sense of cosmic unity. Psychiatrist Stan Grof described basic characteristics of the cosmic unity experience as "transcendence of the subject–object dichotomy, exceptionally strong positive affect (peace, tranquility, serenity, bliss), a special feeling of sacredness, transcendence of time and space, experience of pure being, and a richness of insights of cosmic relevance."[98] Though he was referring to the experience of LSD subjects, cosmic unity—or "oceanic ecstasy," as Grof sometimes called it—was a prevalent descriptor in *Spiritual Midwifery* birth stories. "We were riding the rushes like a surfer rides the waves," wrote Edward of his wife's labor. "The energy would swell up and Janet's eyes would grow deeper until it seemed like I could look through them like peepholes, and see the vastness of the cosmos out beyond her pupils; endless space."[99] Ellen "experienced a whole other level of consciousness that seemed eternal and timeless" during her labor. "Laying there, I felt One with everyone in the Universe."[100] Another experienced a sense of cosmic unity after her daughter was born. "Her eyes opened right away and it looked like the Universe being unfolded before my eyes."[101]

In the countercultural context, then, childbirth became a community event, a source of spiritual awakening and transcendence, and even a psychedelic experience. It took root in northern California as a natural extension of Stephen Gaskin's teachings. As the practice traveled from the hills of San Francisco to the buses on the Caravan and on to Summertown, Tennessee, it gained new meaning and significance. What started as an experiment in alternative birthing became an established profession, a blending of spiritual theories, trial and error, and medical advice.

But it was far from mainstream. Media coverage and the publication of *Spiritual Midwifery* did put alternative midwifery on the map. More was needed, however, to counteract the claims that what was happening on The Farm was risky and selfish, privileging the desires of the mother over the safety of the child. Alternative birth continued to gain credence through new psychiatric theories.

THE BOX

Stanislav Grof was a medical student working in the psychiatry department at Charles University in Prague when a package arrived one morning in 1956. The box was from Sandoz Pharmaceutical Laboratories in Basel, Switzerland. It wasn't that unusual for pharmaceutical companies to distribute their drugs in the hope that researchers would conduct studies on them. What was special about this package was its chemical contents: LSD-25. Sandoz suggested in a letter in the box that LSD "might be used as a kind of unconventional training tool that would provide psychiatrists, psychologists, students, and nurses the opportunity to spend a few hours in the world of their patients."[102]

On November 13, 1956—St. Stanislav's day—Stanislav Grof swallowed 150 micrograms of LSD as one of the earliest Czech volunteers for such a study. "What happened to me was enormous, and seemed like the beginning of a new life," he said later.[103] Within a few hours of ingesting the drug, his entire conception about the human psyche and the role of psychoanalysis was turned upside down. "I couldn't believe how much I learned about my psyche in those few hours," he recalled. "I was hit by a radiance that seemed comparable to the epicenter of a nuclear explosion." The explosion "catapulted" him out of his body. "At an inconceivable speed my consciousness expanded to cosmic dimensions."[104]

The timing was fortuitous, since Grof was in the midst of an existential crisis. Like many psychiatrists in Europe and the United States in the 1950s, he was inspired by Freudian analysis. Psychoanalytic theory, he believed, offered "seemingly brilliant explanations for a variety of mysterious problems—the symbolism of dreams, neurotic symptoms, the psychopathology of everyday life, insights into religion, sociopolitical movements, art, and many others."[105]

The problem was the disconnect between theory and practice. The results of psychoanalysis were extremely limited, he believed, and took massive amounts of time and money. "I had great difficulty coming to terms with this situation," Grof reflected. "To become a psychoanalyst, one had to study medicine. And in medicine, if we really understand a problem, we are usually able to do something pretty dramatic about it."

He needed evidence. According to psychiatrist Jeffrey Lieberman, past president of the American Psychiatric Association and author of *Shrinks: The Untold Story of Psychiatry*, this has been the Achilles heel of the profession from the start. Did mental illness lie within the mind or within the brain? "Oncologists can touch rubbery tumors, pulmonologists can peer through a microscope at strings of pneumonia bacteria, and cardiolgists have little trouble identifying the yellowish placques of artery-clotting cholesterol," he writes. "Psychiatry, on the other hand, has struggled harder than any other medical specialty to provide tangible evidence that the maladies under its charge even exist."[106]

Grof agreed. Over the next fifteen years he would personally conduct over 2,000 psychedelic sessions, at first in Prague and then at the Maryland Psychiatric Research Institute in Catonsville, Maryland. His observations convinced him that Freud's study of human personality was only the tip of the iceberg. LSD had changed everything, demonstrating the inadequacy of the existing theoretical frameworks to explain human personality. Grof proposed what he called "a new Cartography of the human psyche."

The key came from that little box. LSD was a different kind of drug. It was not causing something, per se. Everyone reacted differently, and the experience could be different every time, for every person. Instead, he argued, LSD was a catalyst for psychological processes. It was not "producing artificial experiences by interacting with the brain. Rather, by increasing the energetic level in the psyche, they were bringing into consciousness the contents from the depth of the unconscious." This offered enormous potential to mental health professionals to develop new therapeutic techniques (such as Gestalt therapy, encounter groups, psychedelic therapy, and what Grof would call "transpersonal experiences").

Thus, at the same time that Stephen Gaskin and his followers were applying psychedelic experiences to new ways of living and birthing in Tennessee, Grof set out to recreate these experiences in a laboratory setting. Though they had similar ideas about the potential of psychedelic drugs, Grof and his colleagues at the Maryland Psychiatric Research Institute went out of their way to appear anything but countercultural. LSD trips took place in a controlled environment (a room inside of the hospital), observed by two professionals—a psychiatrist and an assistant. The subject wore a mask and listened to music intended to enhance and guide the session, which was recorded and then analyzed. Did LSD help the terminal cancer patient coming to terms with death? The alcoholic who couldn't stop drinking? The depressed patient contemplating suicide? The answer, Grof believed, in all of these cases was yes.

The therapeutic implications of this drug discovery was revolutionary, according to its advocates. One didn't need to be an alcoholic or suicidal or dying from cancer to benefit from psychedelic therapy. One could simply reach a higher state of consciousness (as the hippies promoted), experience "self-actualization" (as psychologist Abraham Maslow promoted), and could realize his or her highest human potential. Everyone stood to benefit. New conferences and publications in the late 1960s laid the foundation for a "new interdisciplinary approach to the study of consciousness."[107] These ideas solidified into a new form of psychology known as "transpersonal psychology," marked by the introduction of the new *Journal of Transpersonal Psychology* launched by Maslow in 1969.[108]

MAKING THE INVISIBLE VISIBLE: THE MPRI STUDY

Simply put, LSD helped to put psychiatry back in the playing field. "If we accept the basic premise, that psychedelic drugs make it possible to study the content and dynamics of the unconscious processes that are difficult to reach with less powerful techniques," Grof proposed at an anthropology conference in 1972, "the heuristic value of these substances becomes immediately obvious." Psychedelic drugs "exteriorize[d] otherwise invisible phenomena and processes," and in the hands of researchers, they carried "unusual potential as research tools for exploration of the human mind." Here, he believed, is how it would save psychiatry: "It does not seem inappropriate to compare their potential significance for psychiatry and psychology to that of the microscope for medicine or the telescope for astronomy."[109] LSD provided the "tangible evidence" (in the words of psychiatrist Jeffrey Lieberman) that psychiatrists had been lacking since the birth of their profession.

From 1970 to 1975, Stan Grof and his colleagues at the Maryland Psychiatric Research Institute conducted an LSD Professional Study and Training Program: 108 mental health professionals volunteered to serve in the study, both to contribute to psychiatric studies promoting LSD's therapeutic potential and to receive training in order to use it on their own clients. The majority of the subjects were male (86) and the average age was between thirty-nine and forty-one. This was a highly educated group; two-thirds had either an MD or a PhD. The results of the study showed that two-thirds of the subjects had experienced "peak experiences" while under the influence of LSD and noted that these experiences had long-term positive effects. Subjects were asked to write up a description of each treatment immediately after, and then a follow-up report six months, one year, and two years after. Ultimately, however, the researchers were unable to conclusively state any statistically significant long-term trends from the drug—and the study was largely forgotten.[110]

At the time, however, the reports from the subjects proved invaluable to Grof for their articulation of the psychedelic experience in a controlled environment as research for the mainstreaming of psychedelic drugs for therapeutic intervention. Their colorful descriptions appeared to follow a coherent structure that led Grof to develop a new psychological schematic.

Nearly all subjects experienced a fluidity between their bodies and their environment. "The first thing I noticed," wrote Subject 7, a thirty-nine-year-old male, "was a dissolving of some of my body boundaries as I experienced my hands, when placed on top of one another, melt into each other."[111] Subject 6, a twenty-four-year-old male, wrote that "it was like I was slipping through the spaces between cells, the spaces between muscle fiber out into the universe. At one point I remember feeling like a great weight was pressing on my physical body and crushing me and I was leaking out of my body."[112] Subject 15, a thirty-year-old male, remarked that "my body, meanwhile, was moist and felt malleable, as though its boundaries were only arbitrary."[113]

More dramatic was the description of "peak" experiences under LSD (reported by two-thirds of all subjects). "I pushed and pushed and then it was here," wrote Subject 10, a female. "Clear light all about and pure energy . . . not electrical energy but some other kind of energy . . . energy of which I too was composed."[114] Subject 15 wrote, "I was conscious of being stretched out and feeling elongated suddenly and instantaneously a silent wail came from very deep inside almost below me and rushed through me so strongly, so rapidly, that I became a cylinder but as the anguish poured through it brought with it a tremendous surge of energy that shot me skyward but carried me with it. My anguish became my energy that became my joy."[115]

What Grof realized from his own observations and his analysis of these written reports is the striking similarity between these accounts and those of childbirth. "The general idea came fast—but the details were added over the years," he explained. "Searching for a simple, logical, and natural conceptualization of this fact, I was struck by the astounding parallels between these patterns and the clinical stages of delivery." What accounted for the similarities, he wondered? "I gradually realized . . . one common denominator: a significant contribution from the trauma of birth."[116]

Subject 18, a thirty-two-year-old male MD, provided Grof with a coherent and convincing account of the relationship between birth trauma and peak LSD experiences. He received his first dosage (300 mcg; a fairly large dose) on November 21, 1972. Three months later, he was given an even higher dose of 400 mcg. "I began a very strong definite feeling of being in a birth situation and feeling that in order to go through with it," he described after his first session, "I could not use myself but that I had to rely on Stan as the midwife. He would help me through this experience of birth."[117]

This analogy of Grof as midwife must have struck him as a useful and powerful metaphor. By guiding the subject through the memory of birth trauma in a gentler setting, he could help him reintegrate the painful experience and begin to heal.[118] Grof began to realize that, like a spiritual midwife, he could empower his patient to turn pain and fear into something blissful and meaningful and productive.

Subject 18 continued to articulate the significance of birth to human development experienced in his psychedelic trip. "Then I begin to feel my birth as being something important . . . wanting it to be something special, but instead I am perceiving myself being reborn like into a machine or into a space capsule. I feel a coldness about the birth in terms of the mechanical machine quality of it in relationship to glorious noble birth that I would expect."[119] This was, of course, the very assessment of birth reformers who labeled hospital birth as cold and mechanical.

Rather than focus only on the experience for the laboring mother, Subject 18 also underscored the importance for the child. As a mental health provider interested in human behavior, he experienced a revelation regarding the impact of birth and bonding: "I suddenly felt the tremendous importance for the child to have proper love and maternal care after birth. . . . If the child were to be deprived of proper care, the feeling of loss and despair he might have experienced in the womb at birth would have been reinforced throughout his life. He would grow to feel insecure with feelings of doubt and a sense of deep guilt and unworthiness about himself and he wouldn't know why."[120] Ensuring a positive birth experience that enabled an infant to bond with the mother, he suggested, was crucial for human development.

BACK TO BIRTH: GROF'S BASIC PERINATAL MATRICES (BPM)

Grof was sold on this notion. "I started seeing that there was this deep perinatal pool of difficult emotions and physical feelings in the human unconscious, which is the source of various forms of psychopathology . . . roots [of disorders] can be traced to the trauma of birth and difficulties of prenatal life."[121] He created a template of four "basic perinatal matrices" related to the development of the fetus and the experience of birth. These four matrices corresponded roughly to the development of the fetus, followed by stages of labor. Each matrix, Grof argued, had an enormous impact on the

BASIC PERINATAL MATRICES

	BPM I	BPM II	BPM III	BPM IV
RELATED PSYCHOPATHOLOGICAL SYNDROMES	schizophrenic psychoses (paranoid symptomatology, feelings of mystical union, encounter with metaphysical evil forces, karmic experiences); hypochondriasis (based on strange & bizarre physical sensations); hysterical hallucinosis and confusing daydreams with reality.	schizophrenic psychoses (elements of hellish tortures, experience of meaningless "cardboard" world); severe inhibited "endogenous" depressions; irrational inferiority and guilt feelings; hypochondriasis (based on painful physical sensations); alcoholism and drug addiction.	schizophrenic psychoses (sadomasochistic and scatological elements, automutilation, abnormal sexual behavior); agitated depression sexual deviations (sadomasochism, male homosexuality, drinking of urine & eating of feces); obsessive-compulsive neurosis; psychogenic asthma, tics and stammering; conversion & anxiety hysteria; frigidity & impotence; neurasthenia; traumatic neuroses; organ neuroses; migraine headache; enuresis & encopresis; psoriasis; peptic ulcer.	schizophrenic psychoses (death-rebirth experiences, messianic delusions, elements of destruction and recreation of the world, salvation and redemption, identification with Christ); manic symptomatology; female homosexuality; exhibitionism.
CORRESPONDING ACTIVITIES IN FREUDIAN EROTOGENIC ZONES	libidinal satisfaction in all erotogenic zones; libidinal feeling during rocking & bathing; partial approximation to this condition after oral, anal, urethral or genital satisfaction and delivery of a child.	oral frustration (thirst, hunger, painful stimuli); retention of feces and/or urine; sexual frustration; experiences of cold, pain and other unpleasant sensations.	chewing & swallowing of food; oral aggression & destruction of an object; process of defecation & urination; anal & urethral aggression; sexual orgasm; phallic aggression; delivering of a child, statacoustic eroticism (jolting, gymnastics, fancy diving, parachuting).	satiation of thirst & hunger pleasure of sucking; libidinal feelings after defecation, urination, sexual orgasm or delivery of a child.
ASSOCIATED MEMORIES FROM POSTNATAL LIFE	situations from later life where important needs are satisfied, such as happy moments from infancy & childhood (good mothering, plays with peers, harmonious periods in the family, etc.) fulfilling love romances; trips or vacations in beautiful natural settings; exposure to artistic creations of high aesthetic value; swimming in the ocean & clear lakes, etc.	situations endangering survival & body integrity (war experiences, accidents, injuries, operations, painful diseases, near drowning, episodes of suffocation, imprisonment, brainwashing & illegal interrogation, physical abuse etc); severe psychological traumatisations (emotional deprivation, rejection, threatening situations, oppressing family atmosphere, ridicule & humiliation, etc.)	struggles, fights & adventurous activities (active attacks in battles & revolutions, experiences in military service, rough airplane flights, cruises on stormy ocean, hazardous car driving, boxing); highly sensual memories (carnivals, amusement parks & nightclubs, wild kicks & parties, sexual orgies, etc.); childhood observations of adult sexual activities); experiences of seduction & rape; in females delivery of their own children.	lucky escape from dangerous situations (end of war or revolution, survival of an accident or operation); overcoming of severe obstacles by active effort; episodes of strain & hard struggle resulting in a marked success; natural scenes (beginning of spring, end of an ocean storm, sunrise, etc.).
PHENOMENOLOGY IN LSD SESSIONS	undisturbed intrauterine life; realistic recollections of "good womb" experiences; "oceanic" type of ecstasy; experience of cosmic unity; visions of Paradise; disturbances of intrauterine life; realistic recollections of "bad womb" experiences (fetal crises, diseases and emotional upheavals of the mother, twin situation, attempted abortions; cosmic engulfment; paranoid ideation; unpleasant physical sensations ("hangover"); chills & fine spasms, unpleasant tastes, disgust, feelings of being poisoned) association with various transpersonal experiences (archetypal elements, racial & evolutionary memories, encounter with metaphysical forces, past incarnation experiences, etc.)	immense physical & psychological suffering; unbearable & inescapable situation that will never end; various images of Hell; feelings of entrapment & encagement (no exit); agonizing guilt & inferiority feelings; apocalyptic view of the world (horrors of wars & concentration camps, terror of the Inquisition; dangerous epidemics; diseases; decrepitude & death, etc); meaningless & absurdity of human existence; "cardboard world" or the atmosphere of artificiality & gadgets; ominous dark colors & unpleasant physical symptoms (feelings of oppression & compression, cardiac distress, flushes & chills, sweating, difficult breathing).	intensification of suffering to cosmic dimensions; borderline between pain & pleasure; "volcanic" type of ecstasy; brilliant colors; explosions & fireworks; sadomasochistic orgies; murders & bloody sacrifice; active engagement in fierce battles; atmosphere of wild adventures & dangerous explorations; intense sexual orgiastic feelings & scenes of harems & carnivals; experiences of dying & being murdered; religious involving bloody sacrifice (Aztecs, Christ's suffering & death on the cross, Dionysos, etc); intense physical manifestations (pressures & pains, suffocation, muscular tension & discharge in tremors & twitches, nausea & vomiting, hot flushes & chills, sweating, cardiac distress, problems of sphincter control, ringing in the ears).	enormous decompression, expansion of space, visions of gigantic halls; radiant light & beautiful colors (heavenly blue, golden, rainbow, peacock feathers); feelings of rebirth & redemption; appreciation of simple way of life; sensory enhancement; brotherly feelings; humanitarian & charitable tendencies; occasionally manic activity & grandiose feelings; transition to elements of BPM I.; pleasant feelings can be interrupted by umbilical crisis: sharp pain in the navel, loss of breath, fear of death & castration, shifts in the body, but no external pressures.
STAGES OF DELIVERY	BPM I.	BPM II.	BPM III.	BPM IV.

Figure 3.6 Stanislav Grof, Basic Perinatal Matrices chart, MSP 1, Box 16, Folder 1, from Purdue University Libraries. Reprinted by permission.

human psyche. "Thinking in terms of the birth," he explained, "provides new and unique insights into the dynamic architecture of various forms of psychopathology and offers revolutionary therapeutic possibilities."[122] But more was at stake than simply recovery of unconscious traumas in birth.

Under the right conditions, he argued, these processes could lead to "orgi-astic feelings of cosmic proportions, spiritual liberation and enlightenment" along with "mystical union with the creative principle in the universe."[123]

The similarity in language and descriptions between LSD peak experiences in the laboratory and spiritual birth on The Farm cannot be overlooked. They appear to be describing almost exactly the same thing. It might seem surprising to see these unexpected entanglements between psychedelic psychiatry and spiritual midwifery. Yet both psychedelic psychiatrists and spiritual midwives benefited from this ideological overlap.

For the midwives, Grof's findings added to their belief that an out-of-hospital birth was beneficial to the baby and not just empowering to the mother. Frequently accused of being irresponsible and selfish by choosing to stay out of the hospital, home birth mothers and their midwives wel-comed evidence that implied psychological benefits to the baby.[124] They believed that what they were doing was not only spiritual and countercul-tural but scientific, and they drew upon not only a midwifery manual written in communist China, but also the theories of scientists—including psychedelic researchers—to buttress their claims. The end result, in the form of a book such as *Spiritual Midwifery*, was a growing acceptance and mainstreaming of out-of-hospital birth.

For the psychiatrists, the connection between psychedelic "peak experiences" and spiritual birth further legitimized their claims that psycho-active drugs offered insights into human behavior and consciousness. Like midwives, psychedelic psychiatrists were wary of being labeled as irrespon-sible or hedonistic. By marketing LSD as a therapeutic research tool that could heal wounds from traumatic birth, they positioned their craft as cut-ting edge. Both groups—the midwives and the psychedelic researchers—borrowed from each other's belief systems and theories to legitimize their own claims about the significance of awakening the unconscious. By doing so, they expanded the parameters of their professions, suggesting the possi-bility of new approaches to the psychology of the mind and the psychology of birth.

CHAPTER 4

⌀

The Bowland Bust

Medicine and the Law in Santa Cruz, California

In the spring of 1974, three women were arrested in an undercover sting operation in Santa Cruz, California, and charged with practicing medicine without a license for their involvement in out-of-hospital births coordinated by the Santa Cruz Birth Center. Over a period of nearly three years, the case moved from the district to the state supreme court, which ruled that pregnancy was a physical condition and that the law prohibited unlicensed persons from "diagnosing, treating, operating upon or prescribing for a woman undergoing normal pregnancy or childbirth." The decision was clearly a blow to unlicensed lay midwives, as well as pregnant women who sought their care. Over the next fifteen years, some forty to fifty midwives were prosecuted in California. "We were the prosecution capital in the U.S.," one midwife argued.[1]

Coverage of the Santa Cruz Birth Center bust put midwifery back on the map, generating a widespread national debate about childbirth, medicine, and the law. One Santa Cruz midwife recalled, "after the bust, there was tremendous support from everywhere, everywhere. People were giving money. People were putting in energy. People were really concerned. People without children—old people, young people. Lots of different kinds of people, which was really impressive, really impressive."[2] An article in *Rolling Stone* magazine noted that just two months after the arrests, the Santa Cruz midwives had "won celebrity status of a sort within national women's health circles." Assistant District Attorney William Kelsay was flooded with hundreds of angry letters protesting the arrests. Health feminist Sheryl Ruzek noted that "the lay midwives and their clients, with all

95

their traditional values, came to be viewed as warriors in the feminist battle for freedom of choice."[3]

These women became further venerated in print and on film. Journalist Suzanne Arms included a chapter on the Birth Center midwives and the bust in her 1975 bestseller *Immaculate Deception*, and in 1985, Impact Productions released *Push: A Women's Western* featuring Suzanne Arms, Raven Lang, and Kate Bowland discussing the arrest and their decision to become "pioneer" home birth midwives. As the story of the Birth Center bust evolved, and in each retelling, it carried great symbolic weight—a testament to the enormous divide between midwifery and medicine and to conflicting beliefs about where and how childbirth should take place.

Though they served a purpose, none of these versions of the Birth Center bust capture the nuance and complexity of what actually happened on the ground. The symbolism of the resulting legal case, which pitted midwives against organized medicine and the law, flattened perceptions of a dynamic and collaborative enterprise in ideas and practice in northern California. The story has been buried under the weight of legal analyses, reproductive politics, and media coverage. *Bowland v. Municipal Court*, which established a precedent of state restrictions over parental choice in childbirth options, suggested the near impossibility of unifying reproductive rights groups under the larger rubric of "choice."[4] This chapter narrates the story of the Santa Cruz Birth Center bust and the players involved in order to analyze the potential for collaboration between midwives and doctors, feminists and back-to-the-landers, politicians and activists—as well as the obstacles that ultimately prevented them from doing so.[5]

THE BUST

At approximately 10 a.m. on Wednesday, March 6, 1974, midwives running the Santa Cruz Birth Center received a telephone call from the husband of a client who had ostensibly gone into labor at her rustic cabin in Ben Lomond, California. Wednesdays were "clinic day," the one day of the week when pregnant women came to the center for collective prenatal care. Midwife Kate Bowland stayed behind with her pregnant clients, sending midwife Linda Bennett and apprentice Jeanine Walker on the call. When they arrived at the cabin, with Bennett's toddler in tow, they expected to find client Terry Johnson huffing and puffing away.

"But it didn't look like anybody lived there," Bennett recalls. There were a few people in the house, but no sign of a laboring woman. Someone assured Bennett that Johnson was in the shower, and hearing the water running in another room, the midwives set their birth kits down and assessed the situation. Bennett began to suspect something was off when she opened the refrigerator and found it empty. She checked the cupboards and they, too, were bare. She went to the bed and discovered it was short sheeted. "And that's when somebody shoved money into my hands."[6] Jeanine ran toward the bathroom to see if Terry Johnson was really in the shower, but a woman sprang in front of her and blocked her from entering.

Moments later, a "motley assortment of state investigators, sheriff's deputies, and DA's men poured into the cabin."[7] Assistant District Attorney Bill Kelsay, who would later serve as prosecutor in the case, recalled that the scene was "hilarious. . . . nobody said anything. The women must have wondered what the hell was going on. So finally the sheriff and I said, 'Will someone please tell the ladies what's happening?' "[8] The women were questioned, their birth kits confiscated, and even Bennett's daughter's diaper was searched. "I really hoped she'd pooped but she hadn't," Bennett later laughed. Within thirty minutes of entering the cabin, Bennett and Walker were arrested and charged with practicing medicine without a license. "I remember saying to them defiantly, 'do you think this is going to matter? Do you think this is going to make any difference?' "[9]

The arrests did not spring up out of the blue. The State Department of Consumer Affairs and the Board of Medical Examiners were well aware of the growing presence of unlicensed women assisting women with home births, whose primary qualification consisted of attending other home births. The state of California had stopped issuing midwifery licenses in 1949, and only three aging certified licensed midwives still remained by the time of the arrests twenty-five years later, according to Linda Bennett. Despite this, the number of registered home births increased by nearly fifty percent between 1967 and 1972; these numbers may have been significantly higher, as many home births went unreported.[10] Legally recognized midwifery had virtually disappeared in the state, but had recently been replaced by a handful of young women determined to reclaim home birth as a civil right.

Unlike the underground movement of abortion activists at the time, these women did not try to hide what they were doing. Fliers, conferences, and the publication of Raven Lang's *Birth Book*, a graphic manual of home births taking place in Santa Cruz, publicized their actions. "Because of the system," wrote Lang in the introduction of her book, "midwifery as practiced in this book is against the law . . . we have become criminals."[11] Although Bennett later recalled fear, confusion, and anger at her arrest, it was hardly a surprise.

Back at the Birth Center and unaware that her colleagues had been arrested, Kate Bowland continued to see her clients. She shared a home, a 2,600-square-foot house built in 1873, with a few others, but on

Wednesdays it was filled with pregnant and postpartum women, sharing advice and stories as midwives measured fundal heights. March 6th started out no differently. Paula Miller was there showing off her two-week-old infant, born at home after a twenty-hour labor. "We were sitting and chatting when suddenly there was a mad rush," she remembered. Bowland looked out the window and saw eight cars pull up in front of the house. Assistant DA Kelsay was joined by two other men from the DA's office, members of the sheriff's department, the Santa Cruz city police, and officers from the State Department of Consumer Affairs, including the man who had posed as the pregnant woman's husband. "I sprang to my feet," Bowland remembers, "grabbed the medical contents of my birth kit, Pitocin, syringes, sutures and Xylocaine and plunged them deep into the pocket of my mother's black velvet coat in my closet."[12] Miller recalled that "men with anxious expressions came running round the back of the house. Some more came through the front door with search warrants and roamed all over the house. One of them threw back his coat to show off his gun. I went running over to pick up my baby."[13] Officers searched the house and confiscated

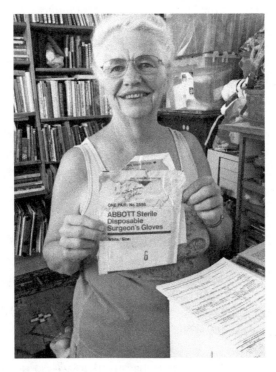

Figure 4.1 Kate Bowland holding a pair of sterile disposable surgeon's gloves, taken as evidence during the bust and then later returned to her. Photograph by Wendy Kline, August 7, 2011. Reprinted by permission.

blood pressure cuffs, stethoscopes, sterile gloves, birth charts, diapers, and a small bag of marijuana. No one was allowed to leave as they conducted their search.

The scene unfolding inside the Birth Center quickly drew media attention. The drama was enhanced by the appearance of two officers in hippie attire, much to the puzzlement and amusement of witnesses. Carol Bredsel, a registered nurse who was in the house during the raid, described the disguises as "really hysterical. I don't know why they wore those hippy clothes. I told the guy, 'your beads are getting caught in your beard.'"[14] Linda Bennett reflected, "it's as if you decided to dress as a hippie and you only had Woolworth's."[15] If the disguises were intended to allow officers to blend in with the clientele (nearly all women and children), it surely

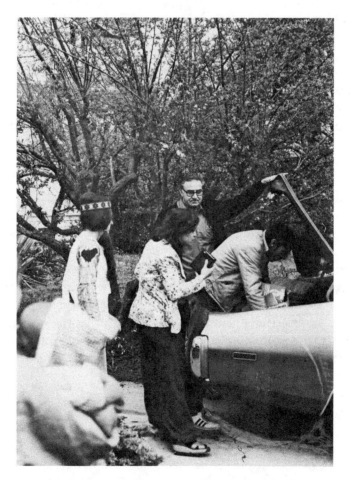

Figure 4.2 Photo of undercover agents at the Santa Cruz Birth Center bust loading evidence into the trunk of their car while being questioned by a reporter. Bowland personal collection.

failed, underscoring the divide between the local counterculture and law enforcement.

Birth Book author and Birth Center founder Raven Lang, who had left Santa Cruz for Vancouver a few months earlier, was temporarily back in town and had intended to visit the Birth Center that afternoon. Unaware of what had taken place, she phoned Bowland to tell her that she would be stopping by. "She told me that there were a ton of cops in plain clothes roaming through her house, looking for some kind of contraband," Lang remembers. "I was very clear and asked her if this was a bust in the making and Kate replied that it was and that as we spoke men were going through everyone's stuff with a fine-toothed comb. So I told Kate I was going to hang up, call the newspapers and the local radio stations, get them down there, and I was on my way." She made the calls, and KUSP radio station, *Sundaz*, and *Santa Cruz Times* reporters quickly joined the confused scene. "The place was swarming with folks," she recalled.[16] One reporter pulled out a tape recorder to capture Bowland's voice shouting from the window, delivering a dramatic play-by-play of the events unfolding within.[17] Lang stood hidden among the bystanders watching from the outside. It was a cold day, she recalled, and she was wearing a checkered coat with a high collar and her hair wrapped up in a knitted cap.

According to Lang, some of the officers came outside and began questioning bystanders, showing them a photo of Lang and referring to her as "the ringleader." "I was RIGHT THERE IN THE MIDDLE OF THE CROWD, and one after another policeman came right up to me and asked folks around me and even *me* if I had seen the person in the photo. When I actually saw my face in the photo and looked into the eyes of the cop, I laughed a little in my mind, while negating my head and saying 'nope, never saw her before' and they just walked onto the next person."[18] Lang remained on the scene, and eventually Kate Bowland was brought out in handcuffs. A photographer captured Kate walking across the lawn flanked by a police officer and a reporter. Bowland smiles triumphantly at the camera, while the officer averts the camera's lens, looking downward as if caught in a criminal act. If Bennett doubted whether the arrest was going to make a difference, Bowland appeared confident that it would.

Lang and other supporters lost no time in organizing. "Oh God, it was an exciting time," she recalls. A law school friend of hers helped her find a large meeting space in a community building later that evening, where "tons of folks" showed up to strategize. "People were bursting the walls apart.... we were all so idealistic, sure that we would change the course of birth and of women's place in it, and that we would find a lawyer for us, finally, and tell the community at large, and the state of California just what we planned to do and why."[19]

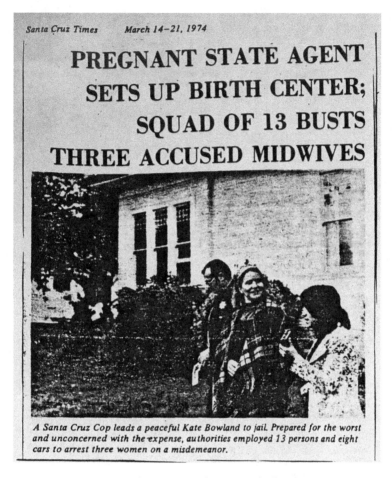

Santa Cruz Times   March 14–21, 1974

PREGNANT STATE AGENT SETS UP BIRTH CENTER; SQUAD OF 13 BUSTS THREE ACCUSED MIDWIVES

A Santa Cruz Cop leads a peaceful Kate Bowland to jail. Prepared for the worst and unconcerned with the expense, authorities employed 13 persons and eight cars to arrest three women on a misdemeanor.

Figure 4.3 *Santa Cruz Times*, March 21, 1974. Bowland personal collection.

As the drama moved from the Birth Center to the courtroom, it assumed greater meaning. It was "the ultimate test case," reflected one supporter of the midwives. "It had to happen sooner or later." Was birth a medical event that required the supervision of an obstetrician in a maternity ward, or a spiritual ritual whose location and procedure should be decided by the laboring woman? Were these young self-appointed lay midwives irresponsible quacks defiantly practicing something for which they had received no training, or were they victims of a misogynist legal system that had robbed spiritual healers of their rightful place in the birthing room? Decided in a court of law, there was little opportunity for nuance. They were either guilty or innocent of violating section 2141 of California's Business and Professional Code. Initial attempts to dispute the charge by claiming there were not sufficient legal grounds to justify legal action failed. The polarizing

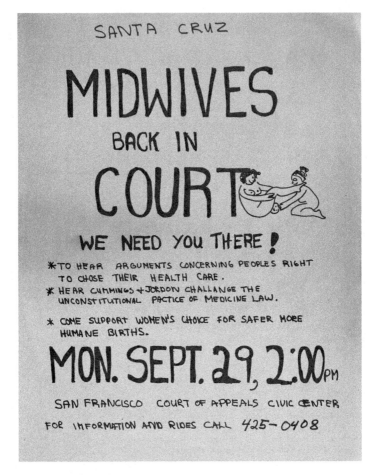

Figure 4.4 One of many handwritten fliers demonstrating the active role of midwifery supporters during the Bowland case. Bowland personal collection.

effects of the courtroom reaffirmed the assumption that midwifery and medicine did not mix.

The media and the midwives of California crafted a particular public image that, after the arrest, glossed over their connections to medicine. Examining who these women were and why they came to identify as midwives in the early 1970s reveals a more complex portrait of California counterculture and women's changing relationship to medicine. The police had targeted Raven Lang as the ringleader because she had started the Birth Center and had published the controversial *Birth Book*. Though she chose to keep a low profile at the time of the bust, she fearlessly catalyzed the events leading up to it.

"BORN A FEMINIST": RAVEN LANG AND THE CREATION
OF THE SANTA CRUZ BIRTH CENTER

"I think I was born a feminist," Lang reflected in 1986. "I was born wanting to be heard." A sickly child, she suffered from asthma, polio, and rheumatic fever, hospitalized for a year during her adolescence. "Never did I take health for granted."[20] She yearned to study science, but her Catholic school offered her literature instead. Hoping to become a doctor, she was pre-med in college, but dropped out her junior year. Then she discovered a passion for art, which opened her eyes "to another whole way of looking," she recalled. She received a scholarship to study at the San Francisco Art Institute, where she met Kate Bowland. She got married, became pregnant, and quit her studies, supporting herself as an art teacher at a private school.

The birth of her child, she argues, changed the course of her life. She was twenty-five years old in 1968, and she and her husband could not afford a private obstetrician, so they opted for a $350 package deal offered by Stanford University Hospital that covered prenatal appointments and a hospital delivery. She read everything she could on natural childbirth—Grantly Dick-Read's *Childbirth without Fear* (1945) and Marjorie Karmel's *Thank You, Dr. Lamaze* (a personal account credited with introducing and popularizing the Lamaze method to the United States in 1959)—and optimistically awaited labor. When contractions began, she stayed at home as long as possible, and arrived at the hospital already halfway dilated. "And so I labored for about four hours and then they basically gave me an episioproctotomy in order to get him out because it was a very busy night and they had to move people in and out of the delivery room," she remembers.[21] As soon as the baby was born, he was taken away from her and put in a nursery, despite her pleas to hold him. Like many women in the late 1960s and early 1970s who spoke out against hospital birth experiences, Lang believed that the treatment she received was not in the best interests of her or her baby. "In retrospect, some of the deepest pain that I have was in that fact that I was so bewildered by what they did to me, so bewildered and so insulted, that my instincts at that time betrayed me. I didn't say to them, 'You motherfuckers! You get out of here. This is my kid.' I didn't even know how to use that word at the time."[22]

When Lang returned home from Stanford Hospital two days after the birth, she found a strong desire to talk to people about what had happened to her. "I kept wanting to uncover it—you know, look underneath all the rocks—turn over every rock because something didn't make sense to me. And there was nobody to talk to."[23] Lang felt completely isolated as a young mother. She did not know many other women with children and had never seen a woman breastfeed. "It was a different world," Lang recalls, "when you think about how different birth practices and customs are in such a short time, in just one adult's life span. You know, when I went to my last post-partum visit at Stanford I went with a series of questions that the physician couldn't answer, and I then realized that my experience in birth would lead me on a journey that I would have to delve into and figure out for myself."[24]

She went on a quest for answers. Surrounded by farm animals, her first births were goats with breech births requiring assistance.[25] A few months later, she learned from a friend that there were some women living close by in the Santa Cruz mountains who were helping each other have their babies at home. She told her friend that she wanted to meet these women.[26]

Shortly after, lay midwife Diane Scamzer drove her VW bus on the curvy road that led to Raven's house in Ben Lomond.[27] Raven, who did not identify as part of the counterculture at the time, was astounded by what she saw. "[Diane] was definitely a hippie of the first order," Raven later recalled. Diane carried her little blond boy, the same age as Raven's son, into the house and proceeded to remove her shirt and breastfeed. She told Raven how she gave birth in her own home in Boulder Creek and that she had attended sixteen other home births over the past year and a half.[28] She stayed for hours, then hiked down the road to a house with a telephone to check on a woman in labor. When Raven learned that the woman was ready to deliver, she begged to come along, and Diane consented. "And then when I saw this woman give birth on her own power, every question I had asked in the postpartum visit at Stanford was answered by this woman. I thought, oh my god, this birth compared to mine was like day and night."[29] Witnessing a natural birth in a woman's own home, with no intervention, no haste, and no incisions further confirmed her belief that what had happened during her own delivery was unjust, a cold, sterile parody of a sacred event.

How were women to learn of alternatives to hospital birth? No childbirth education classes existed in the area.[30] Raven decided she would fill that gap, posting notices or classes in local laundromats and food co-ops. Though she did not have a phone or any way for interested couples to respond, she waited expectantly in her living room on that first day. When six couples showed up at the appointed time, she took it as an indicator that this "was the beginning of my career in birth."[31]

Raven spent the next few years teaching and participating in births, some in hospitals, some at home. The first time a young pregnant woman asked Raven to be her midwife, she said no. "I had a lot of sobriety about the birth process; there were many things that could happen that I wasn't trained to do."[32] Lay midwife Diane had moved away, just as local interest in home birth was growing, leaving a dearth of practitioners. Still, Raven was hesitant, believing that "there was a big part of [Diane] that was quite uneducated and there was a part of me that never quite got behind all that. I couldn't just trust it all to be groovy. I knew that at some point it wouldn't be groovy and someone was going to need some emergency procedures or some sort of knowledge this woman didn't possess."[33] She wanted to know more about the mechanics of birth, but there were very few books available, other than standard obstetrical textbooks and *Thank You, Dr. Lamaze* and *Childbirth without Fear*. As the authors of *Our Bodies, Ourselves* were discovering in Boston in these same years, much of the material on reproduction and women's bodies needed to be written by participants in the movement. Until the publication of *The Birth Book* in 1972 and *Our Bodies, Ourselves* in 1973, American readers had almost no access to basic information, images, or personal accounts of women's reproductive experiences.[34]

Though home birth seemed like a reasonable endeavor to Lang, she discovered there was very little support within the medical community. When she approached her psychiatrist friend, Dr. Bob Spitzer, asking if he had any books on obstetrics she might study, he was shocked to learn of the growing interest in home birth. Why would a woman want to have her baby at home, when she could do it in the hospital with a doctor? Perhaps, he thought, "these women could be just another variety of California 'kook.'" He sought these women out, hoping to dissuade them, but discovered that they all had remarkably similar stories. "They were not 'kooks,' but for the most part were intelligent women who were not unaware of the medical danger involved." Clearly a new movement was underway to uncover the potential benefits of home birth to mother and child.[35]

Spitzer became convinced that home birth was a legitimate endeavor, but, according to Lang, he was one of few local doctors who supported the cause. One general practitioner, Peter Nash, had been attending home births but had been dissuaded by colleagues from continuing the practice. In January of 1971, local obstetricians and public health officials met to discuss the increasing prevalence of home births. Nash and Lang attended the meeting, hoping to enlighten the obstetricians about why more women were making this choice, but because they were not doctors they were not allowed to speak. "As a result," Lang explained, "there was no discussion of philosophical differences, and, ultimately, no understanding."[36] Instead, the obstetricians decided as a group to refuse prenatal care to any woman expressing interest in having a home birth.[37]

For Lang, this refusal was a call to arms. She contacted all the women currently involved in childbirth education or attending home births—she knew of eight other women who were involved by 1971—and invited them to her home.[38] Three of the women were nurses already involved in prenatal care. They talked about strategies and mulled over the idea of joining

forces to more effectively provide services that were increasingly in demand. "Some were scared because it wouldn't be legal," Lang wrote, "and
we'd be up for lots of criticism and a possible bust." Despite this, seven
women decided it was the "only solution. We were already doing it, so there
was no reason why we shouldn't organize and help each other out."[39] They
met regularly, sharing ideas and experiences. "Suddenly we found ourselves
starting our own school, teaching each other and ourselves."[40] The nurses
taught physiology and anatomy. Others discussed moral, political, and social issues.[41]

In March of 1971, the Santa Cruz Birth Center opened its doors in a private home in the center of town. Here, these seven women hoped to spread
the knowledge they had gained on their own to the wider community of
women interested in home birth. "I went to the birth center when I was
four months pregnant, the first day it opened," announced Jan at a seminar held by the Birth Center the following year. "It was the highlight of my
pregnancy because I could go there and hang out with the pregnant ladies."
Jan explained that much of what she learned came from the women who
returned to the center after giving birth, "and she'd give us all the details
about what went through her heart, her mind, her body during the birth,
and all about her fears and complications."[42]

The center provided more than just moral support. The supplies the
founders chose to include at the center suggested the extent to which they
believed pregnancy and birth required at least a certain degree of technology
and medicine. According to Lang, on the first day they were equipped with
"about seven empty charts to fill in, some piss sticks for checking protein
in the urine readings, a blood pressure cuff, a stethoscope, a scale, a stack
of books, photographs, a movie which we had made of a birth, and a whole
lot of energy."[43] Like other women's health organizations that were starting
to crop up across the country, the Birth Center founders were not vehe-
mently opposed to the practice of medicine. They just believed that when it
came to women's reproductive health, lay women were as capable as medical men, if not more so, in practicing it. But medicine was only one aspect
of the birth process, which they viewed as a spiritual rite of passage with
the potential to empower the mother and strengthen the maternal–infant
bond. And these spiritual components, invested with new meaning by perinatal psychology, the counterculture, and women's health movements, had
no place in a hospital birth.

Thus, the Birth Center fulfilled two purposes in Santa Cruz County. On
the practical side, it provided prenatal care to women who believed they
could no longer obtain it from local obstetricians. Workers checked urine,
took blood pressure, and talked about diet and exercise. These were all
procedures that a nurse would do in a medical practice, and some of these

Birth Center workers had nursing licenses. What raised eyebrows and led to the arrest of three of them was the second objective of the Birth Center: to assist women in giving birth at home. The sign they hung on the Birth Center wall stating their philosophy reflected the dual purpose:

> We are a sisterhood concerned with birth and its process. We feel positive attitudes are never too great for the mental, spiritual and physical well being of the child and mother.
>
> We are finding out about natural capabilities of women.
>
> We emphasize the importance of pre and post natal knowledge as well as birth itself. As a birth center we will share our knowledge and love of pregnancy, lactation, and infant care. Classes will be available for instruction in body building exercises, physiological and psychological changes in pregnancy, nutrition, relaxation, breathing, the mechanics of labor and birth, care of the newborn, and related subjects.
>
> We are a group of people who have taken our birthright—freedom, and decided for ourselves what our rituals of birth will be.[44]

Within the first year, some seventy to eighty young women came through the Birth Center, even though its physical location changed four times (perhaps an indicator of their limited budget of $150). Fifty of them gave birth at home that year. Out of these dramatic experiences emerged powerful birth stories. "People would write their birth story and give it to me and I would read it to my next class and I would see the effect," Lang recalled. Sometimes she would invite couples back to the group after they had given birth to recount their experiences. "They would tell the person all about their birth and I would see the effect that it would have. And I would see the effect of a good story vs. a difficult story or a bad outcome. And then I said I'm going to make a book."[45] The information and images were powerful, and she imagined that with the right packaging, the book could change the way people thought about where and how to give birth.

Many, though not all, of the stories Lang chose to include in the *Birth Book* were joyful depictions. "It was a miracle!" exclaimed Linda Sibley of the birth of son Kevin in May, 1971. "I do not think that I will ever in my life experience any one thing more exalting than the birth of our son." While she delighted in sharing the experience with friends and relatives, her real gratitude was for Lang. "I will never forget the image of [Lang] sitting along side of the bed, her warm and beautiful eyes feeding my soul with strength and reassurance, and I knew everything was just right and well." Even Linda's skeptical sister-in-law changed her attitude toward home birth after meeting Raven. "I wish I had met and talked with you before to catch some of your sureness. You gave a calm, capable reassuring impression in spite of being so young."[46]

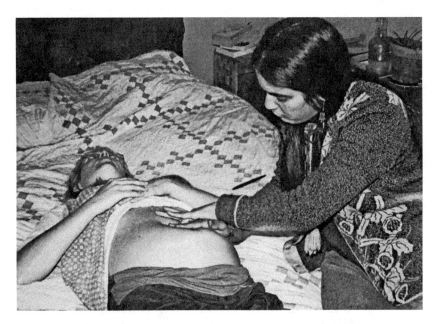

Figure 4.5 Raven Lang examining home birth client, published in *Birth Book* (Felton: Genesis Press, 1972), 5. Reprinted by permission of Raven Lang.

Lang also chose to include birth stories that required medical intervention. Suebi's contractions were strong, five to seven minutes apart, when she called Lang on the evening of June 9, 1971, but Sunshine Benjamin would take another forty hours to be born in his parents' teepee. "I had no fear until I was afraid of going to the hospital," Suebi wrote after she became aware that her labor was not progressing normally.[47] Lang arrived at 2 a.m. and watched her through the night, and psychiatrist Dr. Bob Spitzer arrived at 3:30 a.m. When contractions began to slow late the next morning, Spitzer and Lang went to the store to buy black and blue cohosh, herbs that had been used for centuries to induce or restart a stalled labor. Suebi drank a cup of it brewed with honey and promptly threw it up, and there was blood in the vomit. By late afternoon, Lang did an internal exam and determined that Suebi was 8 cm dilated, but that labor had stalled. That evening, she and Spitzer decided to telephone Dr. Don Creevy, an obstetrician at Stanford University, to ask his opinion. He recommended stripping Suebi's membranes and giving her an enema and a shot of Pitocin. "Back to the teepee," Lang wrote. "We are all worried; the day is over and the second night upon us. Suebi has much less strength." Spitzer headed to the hospital pharmacy to pick up Pitocin, which she administered in three shots in Suebi's upper arm muscle over the next seven hours. Finally, at 9 a.m., Sunshine was born.[48] Though the birth took place in a teepee, it involved many processes associated with hospital rather than home birth. Lang relied on the expertise of obstetrician Creevy and the medical qualifications of psychiatrist Spitzer in order to keep Suebi out of the hospital.

But did the decision to intervene always require a doctor's assessment? Could midwives practice medicine? Lang included another birth story to illustrate the extent to which she and the other midwives struggled with this question. The case involved a pregnant woman with preeclampsia who insisted on having a home birth despite her awareness of the risks involved. When she showed up at the Birth Center in labor and running a fever, the midwives realized the fetus was in the breech position and transported her to the hospital. "When all this came down on us, we realized we were going to have to become more medical," Lang wrote. She convinced her friend Dr. Bob Spitzer to educate them about blood types, pelvic measurements, and other medical information.

But some midwives were not happy with the idea of becoming more medical. Wasn't their whole purpose to reclaim birth as a spiritual, rather than a medical, event? "Soon we were becoming so medical ourselves that we began to hear criticism from the pregnant community," wrote Lang. "They said we had become less sensitive and personal than [in] our beginning days." In other words, they were becoming more like doctors, the very people they had set out to critique. "We were not as involved in their psychological cycles and their needs. They didn't want us to lose these special qualities that we had."[49] Did an increased emphasis on medical aspects of birth inevitably lead to a decline in sensitivity toward laboring women? Was it possible to retain both qualities?

The search for the proper balance between medical, psychological, and spiritual continued to be debated beyond the first year. On March 25, 1972, the Birth Center sponsored a seminar on home birth in Bob Spitzer's large geodesic dome in Ben Lomond. "Even with all the technological advancements of today, obstetrics has left out the psychological, spiritual, and sexual aspects of birth," seminar organizers announced in a flyer advertising the event. "Women all over the country are experiencing a deep disappointment and even shock over their treatment at hospitals." With that in mind, the Santa Cruz midwives announced the need to come together "to discuss and recognize the needs of the childbearing community who thinks differently than the American Medical Association. We can no longer ignore the reality of home birth," they wrote. Their final sentence was strikingly prescient: "Everyone, *doctors and nurses included*, must work together in order to make it as safe and fulfilling as possible."[50] Decades before an organized lay midwifery movement called for such a collaborative model, the Santa Cruz midwives articulated this need to work together with, rather than in opposition to, doctors and nurses. In addition, they made it clear

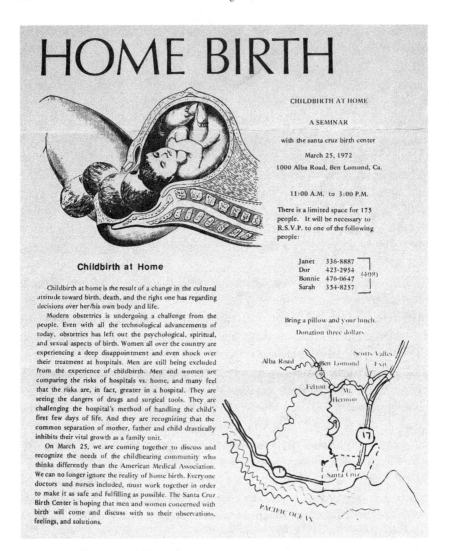

HOME BIRTH

CHILDBIRTH AT HOME

A SEMINAR

with the santa cruz birth center

March 25, 1972

1000 Alba Road, Ben Lomond, Ca.

11:00 A.M. to 3:00 P.M.

There is a limited space for 175 people. It will be necessary to R.S.V.P. to one of the following people:

Janet   336-8887
Dor   423-2954   (408)
Bonnie   476-0647
Sarah   354-8257

Bring a pillow and your lunch.

Donation three dollars

Childbirth at Home

Childbirth at home is the result of a change in the cultural attitude toward birth, death, and the right one has regarding decisions over her/his own body and life.

Modern obstetrics is undergoing a challenge from the people. Even with all the technological advancements of today, obstetrics has left out the psychological, spiritual, and sexual aspects of birth. Women all over the country are experiencing a deep disappointment and even shock over their treatment at hospitals. Men are still being excluded from the experience of childbirth. Men and women are comparing the risks of hospitals vs. home, and many feel that the risks are, in fact, greater in a hospital. They are seeing the dangers of drugs and surgical tools. They are challenging the hospital's method of handling the child's first few days of life. And they are recognizing that the common separation of mother, father and child drastically inhibits their vital growth as a family unit.

On March 25, we are coming together to discuss and recognize the needs of the childbearing community who thinks differently than the American Medical Association. We can no longer ignore the reality of home birth. Everyone doctors and nurses included, must work together in order to make it as safe and fulfilling as possible. The Santa Cruz Birth Center is hoping that men and women concerned with birth will come and discuss with us their observations, feelings, and solutions.

Figure 4.6 Home Birth Seminar flier, March 25, 1972. Bowland personal collection.

that they had two objectives: to make birth as safe as possible, but also ful-filling, an event to be cherished rather than endured. Both aspects were needed.

The geodesic dome was filled to capacity that day, as close to two hundred people traveled from as far as Canada and southern California to attend the four-hour seminar, bringing their $3.00 donations and sack lunches. Scott Frankenberg remembered, "I came spinning away from the seminar with a feeling of high energy that comes when you are in contact with someone or some group whose feelings and thoughts are concentrated and focused positively. . . . For the most part the first half of the day was made up of the smooth energy of personal experiences; women who told of home births spoke of the pleasures, the joy, comforts and fears which encompassed their experience; women who had their children in hospitals talked of their help- less and impotent feelings and the sterility of the situation."[51] Clearly there was communal support and even enthusiasm for home birth as a viable al- ternative to hospital birth.

In the afternoon, the discussion turned to politics and the practice of medicine. Don Creevy was one of the few obstetricians in attendance and also one of the few in the state willing to advise and work with the unlicensed midwives. Creevy attended the seminar with photojournalist Suzanne Arms, who would later capture the Santa Cruz birth bust in her 1975 bestseller *Immaculate Deception*. "I think that what we see here is probably just the tip of the iceberg," he said, referring to the growing in- terest in out-of-hospital birth. "The fact that you are functioning is an in- dication in my mind of an organized medicine that has failed dismally to provide for the needs of a significantly large number of people." Too many doctors, unfortunately, he believed, held a "mechanistic view towards med- icine," emphasizing the patient as a "system of tubes and wires" rather than a human being. But they believe that they are doing exactly what they were trained to do, which is to "take care of the mechanical needs of a functioning human body." The problem, according to Creevy (who acknowledged he was not a particularly "welcomed character" within organized medicine), was that "this is not what medicine is all about."[52]

Creevy still had concerns about the safety of home birth, lamenting the lack of communication between trained doctors and lay midwives. Nonetheless, the widespread practice of home birth attended by these midwives indicated to him that organized medicine had failed and that something needed to change. What was happening in Santa Cruz had the potential to reform medicine, not just to provide an alternative, more traditional setting for birth. Allowing for greater communication and collaboration between doctors and midwives could radically alter the parameters—the very definitions—of medicine. Yet after the Birth Center bust two years later, this type of conversation virtually disappeared from public view, as legal issues created new boundaries.

"I BECAME THE MEDICAL ONE": LINDA BENNETT AND THE HOME PREGNANCY TEST

Seminar organizers also established new connections with locals involved in self-help and abortion activism, as they began to see home birth as part of a larger women's health movement.[53] Linda Bennett volunteered to babysit at the birth seminar and met the midwives for the first time. "I was the source for information on legal abortion in the community at the time," she recalls.[54] "For quite a while before I started attending births I was basically what is now called an abortion doula. So I would talk to people and we would talk about all the options available, they would let me know what they wanted, I would show them what options were there for them and then if they wanted a ride I would pick them up."[55] California governor Ronald Reagan had signed the Therapeutic Abortion Act into law in 1967, legalizing abortions authorized by a hospital committee "that finds the pregnancy will gravely impair a woman's physical or mental health."[56] At the seminar, Bennett realized that the politics of birth were closely linked to those of abortion and that the groups should work together. "I told them what I was involved in," she remembers, "and so they became part of the next self-help group and they learned more about gyn."[57]

Bennett spent the first seven years of her life in southern California before moving to the east coast. Her father's position at Ayerst Pharmaceuticals took the family to a new suburb every two to four years when she was a child. After graduating high school in southern California in 1967, she went to live with an aunt in Kathmandu for ten months, a momentous experience for several reasons. She realized that working with people in other cultures "puts your own experiences and your own assumptions and your own decisions into great relief. [It] really helps you see who you are." She also met a marine and got pregnant.[58]

Bennett returned to the United States to attend college at the University of California Santa Cruz, and gave birth to her first child at nearby Dominican Hospital in 1969. Over the next few years, her own reproductive health would influence her political perspective; she suffered a pelvic infection from an IUD, a tumor on her ovary, and a "Reagan sanctioned abortion where I had to promote why I shouldn't be allowed to stay pregnant to a committee who had to decide the merits of my case." Then a former roommate of hers attended a National Organization for Women conference where Carol Downer demonstrated a gynecological self-exam. Bennett was in awe when she heard about this. "Every time I'd been to the doctor it was all kind of a secret. They made the decisions for me; I had no idea what was going on," she realized. "Then I started in a women's self-help group and it was so mind bogglingly amazing to have truth about me revealed that it became my life's work."[59] Being able to see and understand her own anatomy gave her a sense of authority over her body and its functions. The next step was to help other women make that same discovery.

Bennett realized that she had the capacity to provide answers to one of the most potentially life-changing questions a young woman faced: was she pregnant? Prior to the 1960s, pregnancy tests measuring the level of hCG (a hormone produced by pregnant women) in urine was expensive and unwieldy, requiring the use of laboratory animals. New techniques introduced in the 1960s allowed for more widespread testing in hospitals, doctors' offices, and some health departments. Home pregnancy tests did not receive FDA approval until 1977 and then became available for purchase in drugstores so women could have this moment of discovery at home.[60]

Bennett figured out a way to jumpstart the process, offering women the opportunity to discover whether or not they were pregnant outside of the doctor's office at a time when they could not do it on their own. Medical supply catalogs began to sell tests manufactured by pharmaceutical companies in the early 1970s. The tests included reagent anti-hCG serum along with materials that would allow somewhere between 20 and 100 pregnancy tests per kit.[61] "I was always very willing to walk into a medical supply store and pretend I knew what I was talking about and get stuff done," Bennett explained. In essence, she became a lab technician, adding a urine sample to a test tube that contained antibodies against hCG. As Bennett described, "it had little tubes and you had to mix things and time them and look for a circle to appear." She kept the kits in her refrigerator for several years and offered women both testing and pregnancy options counseling.[62]

Thus, long before Bennett became involved in birth, she was familiar with the mechanics of reproductive medicine. "I grew up in a medical household. I grew up with pharmaceuticals all around and a mother who was a nurse. So none of that stuff was ever foreign to me. I grew up with medical textbooks everywhere. I *loved* to look in the back and look at all the grotesque pictures. So it was just something I was comfortable with." These were qualities that she would bring to the Santa Cruz Birth Center. "That was the big criticism for me for a long time was how medical I was."[63] Despite the presence of the blood pressure cuff at the Birth Center, Bennett remembers that initially it went unused.

Bennett's involvement at the Santa Cruz Birth Center began on the periphery in 1972. At first she attended the Wednesday gatherings, bringing along her daughter and talking about self-help and breastfeeding. Then she started getting invited to births, initially to help with childcare or to take pictures. "I went to about a half dozen births before I decided that home birth was ok." Then one weekend when the regular midwives were out of town, she caught her first baby, and things began to change, both for her and for the center. "Once I got involved in the birth center it really became a different thing than the way it had started. And some of it's my fault," she recalls. "Because one of the gifts I have and one of the banes of my existence is seeing contradictions. And one of the contradictions was people were coming to the birth center because they'd heard about home birth and they wanted it. And so they were coming to find a midwife. And up until that point it was basically women who'd had babies helping women who had babies." An outsider to the community, Bennett brought a more medical perspective to the process. "Now there were whole new elements coming in."[64] Increasing demand and popularity inadvertently affected personnel and procedure at the Birth Center.

The March 1972 seminar and the publication of the *Birth Book* later that year increased the visibility of the Birth Center, leading to a rise in clientele as well as the arrests of Bowland, Bennett, and Walker two years later. None of these three women were among the center's founders, and their involvement marked a new stage in the Santa Cruz home birth movement. It was no longer just friends helping other friends give birth, but consumers with heightened expectations of what the alternative movement could do for them.[65] The group found itself overwhelmed, trying to organize, advocate, teach, learn, and catch babies. Inevitably, philosophical differences emerged, such as those Linda Bennett described. "I became the medical one," she recalled. "So when the character of the birth center started changing from mothers who had made the decision to deliver unassisted with the help of their friends to people like me who came in saying yes, now I want to be a midwife, I want to study midwifery, I want to do this for people, then there's more of a separation between you and the mother . . . so that's when you get into a completely different type of mother looking for a midwife."[66] The center's growing popularity affected its structure, philosophy, and even its clientele.

"I NEVER INTENDED TO BE AN OUTLAW": KATE BOWLAND AND THE PSYCHOLOGY OF BIRTH

Like Bennett, Kate Bowland first became involved in the Santa Cruz Birth Center in early 1972, after the seminar but before the actual publication of the *Birth Book*. Raised in southwestern Wyoming, she spent some time as a young girl accompanying a public health nurse making house calls throughout the county. "I credit her with giving me a vision of home care," Bowland writes, "a taste for adventure, and an understanding that the journey is much of the story."[67] In the mid-1960s, she moved to San Francisco, rented an apartment in the Haight-Ashbury district, and enrolled in the San Francisco Art Institute. After she graduated in 1968, she headed to southern Oregon, where she was living when former classmate Raven Lang contacted her in May of 1971 about her decision to form the Santa Cruz Birth Center.[68]

Bowland was fascinated by Lang's account, as well as the birth photographs she sent along, soon to be published in the *Birth Book*. She remembers that the photos were "stark and graphic, shocking to my Midwestern sensibilities, yet absolutely intriguing."[69] Young women wearing nothing but socks, laboring on their hands and knees on mattresses on the floor, offered quite a contrast to the typical image of a woman giving birth in a lithotomy position, her feet in stirrups, in the hospital. Bowland decided she had to see for herself what Lang was doing. She came to visit in February of 1972 and never left, learning midwifery from Lang and the other local midwives. Later that spring, Bowland displayed some of these birth photographs at a women's liberation booth at a street fair in downtown Santa Cruz. When the owner of Bookshop Santa Cruz asked her to remove the photographs, claiming they were disturbing to some middle-class women, a controversy broke out. Bowland was chastised by the president of the downtown merchants association, who accused her of being selfish and egotistical by showing objectionable pictures that did not have anything to do with the "love the earth" theme of the fair. She retorted that it had everything to do with loving the earth and the positive work that women were doing to make it a better place. Thus, well before her arrest, Bowland demonstrated determination and defiance.

Yet she did not portray herself as a rebel. "I never intended to be an outlaw," Bowland has stressed repeatedly over the decades. It is the title of an autobiographical essay published in 2011, but the claim emerged far earlier, in newspapers covering the arrest and ensuing court cases. In the 1985 documentary *Push: A Woman's Western*, she states it unequivocally, looking directly into the camera. "I never set out to break a law. I wasn't rebelling against anything," she says. She acted out of necessity, explaining, "I was doing what had to be done in the moment." After the arrest, she explains on camera, she remembers sitting in the Santa Cruz County jail in disbelief. "They're charging me with a crime? And I was in disbelief because I went to church and I was president of the youth group and I was a Young Republican and I voted and paid taxes. I didn't set out to be an outlaw." If the media wanted to portray her as a self-righteous politicized hippie intent on challenging the law by provoking arrest, she did her best to counter that with a far more conservative image.

On film, she looks more like a turn-of-the-century "Gibson Girl" than a hippie, dressed in a Victorian blouse, a long skirt, and wearing her hair swept up in a bun. Suzanne Arms and Raven Lang are beside her, also formally dressed, their hair done, and wearing makeup. Arms sits in the center in a rocking chair, engaging the two midwives in relaxed conversation about their experiences. The documentary was filmed in a studio with white walls and floor, but made to appear more homelike with wooden chairs, an oriental rug, and several plants. Interspersed between the dialogue is footage from an actual birth, that of baby Ryan, born at home to ICU nurse Desiree

Condon and husband Vinnie, with Bowland and Lang in attendance. Unlike their studio appearance, Bowland and Lang are in relaxed clothing, sweaty and slightly unkempt, obviously hard at work. Lang maintains eye contact and provides verbal support during the birth, while Bowland is positioned at the foot of the bed, gently guiding baby Ryan's head and body as he makes his way out of the birth canal. Vinnie and a birth assistant (as well as film producer Eric Thierman who captured the event on camera) are also present in the modest bedroom. Viewers are thus exposed to both real-life birth footage and to Bowland and Lang's reflections on midwifery care. Impact Productions marketed the thirty-minute movie, which premiered in San Francisco on October 19, 1985, as an educational film (even providing discussion questions) that "presents midwives as pioneers struggling with an

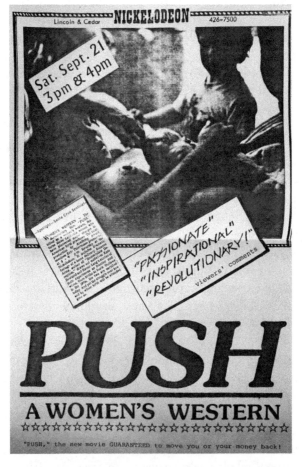

Figure 4.7 Flier for showing of PUSH documentary at Nickelodeon theater, downtown Santa Cruz, September 21, 1985. Bowland personal collection.

outlaw image."[70] The message seems straightforward: these are thoughtful, competent, brave women who have risked a lot—even jail—to serve their community. They did it out of necessity, as a way to preserve and protect a rite of passage that hospital birth did not allow for.

Thus the outlaw image, whether intentional or not, stuck. It raised powerful questions about when and why women lost the right to tend to other women at birth. It also raised awareness of the vulnerability of unlicensed birth practitioners in the United States. But the image, particularly in Bowland's case, also served to mask the much more complex picture of unlicensed midwifery practice in the 1970s. Bowland's early experiences as a midwife, as viewed through her private midwifery journals, correspondence, and unpublished interviews, reveal the extent to which, despite her legal vulnerability, she was politically savvy, educated about medicine, and successful at establishing ties with members of the medical community. Her private reflections sometimes contradicted the public image she put forward in the media. For example, when asked whether she was surprised by her arrest in an unpublished interview in 1987, Bowland answered in the negative. "We were very aware that what we were doing was taboo in our culture, out of the norm, and that the medical establishment was very powerful, very controlling and had essentially eliminated midwifery at the turn of the century. . . . So we were very aware of our political-socio position."[71]

Her journals reveal much more than simply her awareness of the political and legal situation. Her entries from July 1972 to April 1974 (approximately four hundred pages of writing) capture the intense, intoxicating experience that midwifery offered to young idealistic women such as Bowland in the early 1970s. At first glance, Bowland's journals appear as difficult to interpret as those of late eighteenth-century midwife Martha Ballard seemed to be (before Laurel Thatcher Ulrich brought them to life), though the context is quite different. Ballard's diary entries were consistently brief, seemingly filled with trivial detail, and generally devoid of emotion. Bowland's teem with passion and frustration, but are difficult to follow. Meeting notes, addresses and phone numbers, appointments, birth records, poems, to-do lists, scribbles, and sketches appear haphazardly throughout the pages. Lists of books such as "Myths and Falacies in Human Sexuality" [sic] follow notes on preeclampsia and shoulder dystocia in birth, art sketches, handwritten maps to homes, and even notes on the Communist Manifesto. Yet their very haphazardness speaks to the realities of birthing as Bowland experienced it—unpredictable and unique. For example, as she tended to women in labor, she regularly documented pulse, fetal heart tones, and timed contractions. But she also spent a great deal of time waiting and observing, and took advantage of this time to take in her surroundings, compose poetry, make lists, or draw.

During Suzanne's birth on March 18, 1973, Bowland recorded regular contractions between 8:19 and 8:41 p.m. on the left side of the page. To the right of the recorded times, she wrote the following:

> Revolution must come from deep feelings of love.
> Act only on love and trust
> Move forward—obstruction—
> Stop obstruction how best to affect change- educate women
> Don't interfere—let her fight but Jesus how to teach the labor
>   and birth attendants the sensitivity to a laboring woman
>   environment [and] to her physician—she can accept almost
>   anything if explained and reassured -

Until the last few lines, it is not clear whether this piece has anything to do with the laboring mother in the midst of contractions, or why Bowland chose to write it here. But as the entry reveals, this was an emotionally harrowing labor, both for Suzanne and for Bowland. Suzanne had telephoned Bowland that morning to let her know that she was having signs of labor. Bowland came to her house at 12:45 p.m. Two hours later, Suzanne was 2 cm dilated.

At that point, something must have happened, because Bowland's next line refers to an incident in the hospital. "Nurse Glee is awfull," [*sic*] writes Bowland, "-talks and asks questions during a contraction. Argues with her about need to answer. Fills out five papers with medical herstory including abortions." Next, Suzanne refused to let Glee do a vaginal exam. "Glee very unhappy," Bowland continues. "I was asked to get off bed; room getting cooler; hospital very uptight with me." Clearly Bowland senses that Glee resents her support of Suzanne (and perhaps encouragement to refuse a vaginal exam). Yet Bowland interprets this dynamic within the larger context of gender, medicine, and power. She uses passive voice; we don't know whether Glee herself asked her to get off the bed, and Bowland notes that the hospital is uptight with her; not the nurse. "Nurses can not give orders—that [but?] they are sisters. And we are on the same side," she tells herself. "But women must demand their rights. We must acknowledge a laboring woman's need for a quiet supportive environment."[72] Rather than blame Glee, she blames the hospital and the power structure, writing,

> I question everything that a dr. does—the hospital does—in the
>   name of good medical practice –
> Enemas

Vaginal examinations
In and out
Dark labor room
clock opposite the woman
question during admission: abortion/ live births/ marriage/
    baby's name/ breast or bottle

Her frustration with what she witnessed during Suzanne's labor, then, explains what she writes next while recording those 8 p.m. contractions. "Act only on love and trust" and "stop obstruction" are her principles, developed in reaction to hospital protocols that have served to upset and frighten Suzanne, such as having to make mention of previous abortions and receiving vaginal exams.

At 9:06 p.m., shortly after writing these reflections, Bowland notes that Suzanne "had urges to push—very emotional—nurses wouldn't let her push." This undoubtedly added to her frustration that hospital procedure prohibited Suzanne from doing what her body knew to do. The final straw, one of particular concern to the Santa Cruz midwives, was an episiotomy, which they believed to be unnecessary and inhumane most of the time. "10:20 p.m. baby boy born 5 lbs 13 oz 19 inches giant episiotomy," writes Bowland, and then follows with a powerful remark. "Dr. Anzalone looked me in eye as he went to cut her the second time." What was her perception of this gesture? Was this a power play, or perhaps an admonition of guilt? Or simply a recognition on his part that he knew she would disapprove? Nothing in the diary answers these questions.

Bowland proceeds to describe the scenario as one of horror: "Suzanne screams with shot of zilocain [*sic*] and cutting of episiotomy—Anzalone looked very worried as he cut . . ." Bowland suggested that fear or concern might have caused the obstetrician to rush the delivery. She does not reveal the outcome of the birth, but her overall tone is one of frustration at Suzanne's treatment while in the hospital. This was a fairly common sentiment among home birth midwives at the time; after all, many women opted for home births as a result of poor treatment during a hospital delivery or word of mouth about them. Allee Jay and Jade Saxson, two Santa Cruz Birth Center midwives, had both previously worked in hospital maternity wards and attributed their decision to support home birth based on what they had witnessed there.[73]

Despite Bowland's negative reaction to Anzalone's procedures in this 1973 entry, she and other midwives perceived him as more of an ally than an adversary. "He was like the Italian mafia of the OB. He was an obstetrician who was highly skilled and just did his job," Bowland reflected in 2011. He offered to help her whenever she needed it and even lent her obstetrical textbooks. In a prior journal entry, Bowland wrote down "questions for Dr. Anzalone." "Pneumonia in 2nd month; abortion?/ Danger to develop[ment] of fetus/ diet/antibiotics."[74] Presumably she jotted down these notes to remind herself to ask him next time she saw him. Linda Bennett also perceived Anzalone as a supportive obstetrician. "He was wonderful. He was funny too," she recalled, describing him as "maybe 5'5," 5'6" stocky Italian guy." He had taught her to do fundal pressure and was skilled with forceps. "Dr. Anzalone really knew his stuff."[75]

Perhaps even more intriguing is the extent to which Anzalone credited the midwives with changing his birth practices. The *San Francisco Bay Guardian* reported in 1974 that "in Santa Cruz, progress has been made in educating local doctors. Dr. Joseph Anzalone, president of the county medical society, actually changed his methods of dealing with delivering women." Prior to attending a seminar at the Santa Cruz Birth Center, he "made his patients deliver flat on their backs with intravenous tubes in their arms." He did not allow fathers to be present during the birth. "Now his patients have the option of delivering in a sitting position, without drugs, and with company. 'I was beginning to get bored with my practice', he admits, but now his excitement with births has been rekindled."[76]

Anzalone is not the only doctor present in Bowland's journals. Don Creevy, the Palo Alto obstetrician who had spoken at Lang's Birth Seminar in 1972, makes several appearances. When Bowland did a vaginal exam on Tory on April 21, 1973, she realized Tory's baby was in the breech position ("I feel soft fleshy parts like butts and hole") and decided to transport her. At the hospital, Tory was x-rayed, and Creevy determined she would need a C-section. "Creevy told Tory—while touching her face and hands—she really took it well," Bowland writes. Clearly Bowland believed that Creevy's bedside manner reassured the anxious mother. As Bowland had written in the margins next to her recordings of Suzanne's contractions a month earlier, a laboring woman "can accept almost anything if explained and reassured." Yet Bowland was still skeptical of Creevy's decision to do a C-section. "Some part of me really doesn't believe it necessary."[77]

Nevertheless, she relied upon the assistance of obstetricians when problems arose during a home birth. At 11:20 a.m. on March 20, 1973, Bowland arrived at the home of laboring woman Marilyn M., whose contractions were five minutes apart. Bowland described an "air of excitement," where father-to-be Bob Z., two other men, and one woman were "sitting and smoking." The others left, but Bowland and Bob, a psychologist "talked excitedly about his work and our[s] and the similarity in imprinting and attachment."[78]

Raven Lang had written about imprinting and attachment in the *Birth Book*, and Bowland would have been familiar with her argument. Drawing on the work of zoologist Konrad Lorenz and psychiatrist Stan Grof, Lang argued that the birth experience had long-lasting effects on the psychological makeup of the child and the nature of the mother–infant bond. In the hospital, the use of narcotics and the practice of separating the infant after birth could negatively affect the development of this bond and even lead to neuroses later in life. Father-to-be Bob Z., meanwhile, had developed a therapeutic method called "Attachment Therapy" or "rage reduction therapy" to treat attachment disorders by physically restraining the patient. Sometimes this therapy included rebirthing, a re-enactment of a patient's birth trauma as contractions pushed it out of the womb. This theory stemmed from the earlier work of Otto Rank, an Austrian psychoanalyst who theorized that many psychological problems "could be traced back to the trauma of childbirth and the infant's dramatic passage through the vaginal channel."[79]

Bowland may not have known this, but the State Board of Medical Examiners had revoked Bob's license in 1972 after a patient was injured.[80] Despite shared beliefs in the significance of the birth process, Bowland was averse to physical intervention, while Bob promoted it. One can imagine the scenario in which Bowland found herself that day, sitting in the bedroom of a laboring woman, while engaging in an intellectual discussion over psychological theories related to home birth as it was actually taking place.

Only it didn't actually take place that day. Marilyn's labor stalled, and Bowland eventually gave up and went home. She returned at 8:08 a.m. the next morning. "Rained like hell all the way. Contractions modest and Marilyn is in her bed with many pillows—bed facing the corner windows she's looking out into the Santa Cruz mountains—oak, madion {?} red wood fir eucalyptus trees in bloom." Dr. Van Ooy, an obstetrician, came to see her at 9 a.m. and determined she was three centimeters dilated. "He was very reassuring and told her she needed to relax," writes Bowland, though she notes that he did not offer her any drugs to help. "[He] was quite fatherly. Said she had good support."[81] Here was yet another obstetrician who seemed supportive of home birth and the Santa Cruz midwives. He then instructed Bowland to call him at 1:00 p.m. with an update. It appears they were, in a sense, working together.

But Marilyn remained anxious. "She really tensed during an exam," writes Bowland. She spent most of the day and evening laboring on her hands and knees and on her side, with contractions coming every four minutes. Another midwife came to assist Bowland. As labor dragged on, tensions ran high, and the different approaches of psychologist and midwife became apparent. "Bob felt he expected more of us—for us to lock in and 'relax her,'" Bowland noted. "So we began rubbing her legs—forehead arms—talking to her—to relax—she let go and began to fall asleep between contractions."[82]

Like his approach to attachment disorders in children, Bob's approach to birth was clearly more interventionist than Bowland's, and he had no difficulty critiquing Bowland's less invasive method. When she expressed reluctance to do another vaginal exam, "he said I didn't want to do them because I had a 'phallic intrusion complex.'" On the defensive, she "explained the idea of energy forces in relation to vaginas," but then agreed to do the procedure. She noted this exchange twice in her journal entry, undoubtedly a reflection of her frustration.[83] She had become the subject of psychological scrutiny rather than the legitimate provider. Though Bob was supportive of home birth, this scenario indicates the potential conflicts that could emerge between birth provider, a laboring woman, and/or the father of the child. Even within the home birth community, gender, status, and power affected practice and procedure. Out-of-hospital births were not exempt from these established hierarchies, despite attempts to quash them.

After seventeen hours of labor, Marilyn's cervix had only dilated 5–6 of the requisite ten centimeters. By 6 a.m., she had made no further progress, though her waters broke when Bowland examined her again. Bowland called Dr. Van Ooy who instructed her to bring Marilyn to Good Samaritan Hospital. With a fever of 101.6, Marilyn was put in isolation upon their arrival at the hospital. Bowland's notes end there, so presumably she did not witness the actual birth. Like Suzanne's birth before her, Marilyn's ended up far from the envisioned ideal of a peaceful home birth. But the complications allow for a closer view of the varied interactions between midwife, doctor, and family members, hinting at the collaborative work that has been virtually erased from the historic record.

Many of the births recorded in Bowland's early journals do not involve complications and, as a result, tend to be more poetic than practical. On October 25, 1972, Linda C. came to the Birth Center for Wednesday clinic in active labor. When Bowland examined her and discovered her contractions were only three minutes apart, she realized they didn't have much time. Linda lived forty miles away and wanted to deliver at home. At 5:50 p.m. she dove into a "big red funky truck" with Linda in tow. But the drama didn't keep Bowland from poetic observations about the landscape: "We're riding fast now in a red ford pickup—those California golden hills are red and green now after last week's rain. Sunlight, sunset colors are liquid gold—almost gone now—Page Mill Road—narrow hillside super windy. Linda says she is surprised how relaxed she is. Rosy cheeks." They arrived home at 6:20, stopping several times on the bumpy road for her contractions. "Tea is being made. Candles are being lit," Bowland noted. She recorded the time, length, and intensity of the proceeding contractions.

By 6:59, Linda's contractions seemed continuous, and she developed the urge to push. At 7:15 her water broke. By 7:30 the house was filled with visitors, there to witness the 7:42 p.m. birth of a "beautiful boy." "Vibes are beautiful," she wrote, "silence after birth 15 people all one now and slowly someone a woman begins to sing and play the guitar, mother/ father are nude on top—Linda nursing baby—stroking face—looking looking looking at baby—Papa looking looking baby is quiet in mother's arms." Without the guitar and the men, this could almost be a scene from Martha Ballard's late eighteenth-century diary. Penciled in later, she added at the top of the entry, "miracle."

Mara's labor in April of 1973 was similarly peaceful. Bowland and another midwife arrived at 2 a.m. "We are in Ben Lomond mountains," Bowland writes. "Stream and water sounds . . . Redwoods in dark . . . lush and green—clear." Partner Kevin rubbed Mara's back, then hugged her. "Mara is moving around a lot—like a dancer—sitting, rolling lying, during some contractions." She wore a white nightie with a crocheted top, and told Bowland that pushing felt "like multiple orgasms." At 5:01 a.m. their baby boy emerged and opened his eyes right away. Kevin tied and cut the cord. "This is one of the most beautiful labors I've ever seen," Bowland wrote afterwards, making reference to Mara dancing in her white gown and her orgasmic contractions.[84] Bowland's decision to include observations on the natural surroundings and the weather evoke a historic style of midwife accounting (Martha Ballard began almost every diary entry with a statement about the weather). But it also makes sense in the context of the 1970s, when back-to-the-landers, members of the counterculture, and home birthers identified nature and the natural environment as a conduit to sexual and spiritual enlightenment. As Bowland penned in a later entry: "birth is more than a physical act," she writes, "it can be a sexual experience of ecstasy, joy, of family unity, of coming close to the ultimate miracle of life."[85]

The reverse, however, could also be true; poor conditions could negatively affect the experience. In her last recorded birth before the arrest, on March 1, 1974, Bowland noted the bad weather after arriving at Nancy's home at 11:10 a.m. "Day is extremely rainy—drive was full of water falls, tree falls and mudslides in the canyon." The baby's head was engaged in the pelvis and Nancy was having intense contractions. At 12:30, Bowland wrote down the measurement of the fetal heart tones, then noted in parentheses, "just had a talk about money—it is so hard for me to do that—it is somehow embarrassing." Here, we get little sense of the idyllic image of birth so prevalent in other entries. Bowland's perception of the labor may have been negatively affected by her stressful journey and the poor weather, leading her to focus on financial remuneration rather than on the spiritual aspects of the birth, as she usually did.

It is perhaps not surprising, then, that when Bowland learned she was pregnant, nature and the changing seasons played a role in how she wrote about and visualized her developing child. Nature had played a formative role in her own development. When asked later how she was called to midwifery, she responded that "the stars and the river through the desert and the horses and all the critters were my [first] teachers."[86] She composed a poem in her journal in January of 1974, the month with the highest amount of precipitation and the coldest weather in Santa Cruz.[87]

> If things were just a little more simple
> If winter wasn't so just foggy
> I could see my self in this whole thing more gracefully,

she begins the poem, perhaps reflecting some anxiety or frustration about the pregnancy. Yet she is excited about what is growing inside of her.

> Really I am happy, someone has a chance to be born.
> I can't contain the feeling.
> Darkness in winter is infinity
> In its softness—fall has always been my favorite season.
> Where will you be born?
> I love you little fish now your heart just beginning to beat
> And my feet will travel many miles
> Before yours will be seen and everyone you will know. I want
>   for you are the endless days of the summer and the clear
>   clear skies of winter and the space between the start for you
>   to grow.
> I want for you:
> *The space between the stars for you to grow in
> *The sunlight to surround you and illuminate your freedom
> *My love to be light that sunlight
> So come my love and be with me
> K.

Metaphors abound between seasons, love, and growth. Sunlight represents love, and it illuminates freedom. Fall is soft. Her desire to provide her fetus "the space between the stars" to grow in suggests a state of cosmic unity, and what psychiatrist Stan Grof referred to as the "transpersonal realm."[88]

Grof's theories on perinatal experience were influential on both Bowland and Lang; Bowland took notes on his work in her journal shortly after learning she was pregnant, and Lang met and worked with him in the late 1970s. Lang believes Grof profoundly changed the way she approached birth, inspiring her to think outside the box.[89] Grof and the new field of transpersonal psychology bolstered her belief that midwifery-assisted birth could result in profound personal transformation, a message also promoted in Ina May Gaskin's *Spiritual Midwifery.*

Less than three months after Bowland wrote the poem about her pregnancy, she was arrested. Over the next three years, she would "attend more court dates than prenatal visits" and would give birth at home to not just one but two children before the state supreme court issued its decision on her case in 1976.[90] Though she would return to home deliveries just three days after her arrest, her journal overflows with names, addresses, phone numbers, defense committee notes, financial figures, and intense doodling, suggesting a nervous energy as she assessed how to stay out of jail. Her first entry after the arrest begins, "what we going to do!!" While she had consistently been philosophical and reflective in her entries, in the weeks after the arrest she brainstormed more frequently about the meaning of birth and about why she was a midwife. One of her lists reads,

> write:
> Birth
> Herstory
> Bust
> Politics

The rest of the page remains blank, but she makes several attempts to organize her thoughts a few pages later. She begins to write a history of the Birth Center, but stops after a few sentences. Another entry includes notes from a group meeting. "keep it simple," suggests one woman. "get interest." These ideas became more succinct after the Birth Center organized a position statement. "who we are and what we do," Bowland scribbles on one page. "1. share info. 2. educate ourselves/others/each other. we don't heal—nature does. We don't deliver—mothers do. Prevention."[91]

Gradually, Bowland and the other midwives began to craft their public story, simplifying their dynamic roles within birth to one primarily of advocate or supporter rather than practitioner. "We don't deliver babies. We aren't practicing medicine. Women deliver," she writes in her journal in mid-April under the heading "press conference." These notes would make it directly into the official comments of the Defense Committee about a week later.

On April 22, 1974, the Santa Cruz Birth Center Defense Committee issued the following in a press statement:

> I am innocent for I have not committed a crime.
> I do not practice medicine for I am a midwife – not a
>   doctor.
> I do not diagnose – I educate.
> I do not deliver the baby – <u>the mother gives birth</u>
> and the mother or father cuts the cord.
> My role is giving medical information and emotional
>   support to women during pregnancy, labor, and
>   birth—period.

The birth stories contained within Bowland's journals and Lang's *Birth Book* belie this claim; vaginal exams, Pitocin injections, and gently turning the baby's head as it emerges from the birth canal are all indicative of more than mere emotional support. But given that the midwives were charged with practicing medicine without a license, they were forced to either support or refute the claim, and not surprisingly, they opted to refute it. They chose a young feminist attorney in San Francisco named Ann Flower Cumings to represent them (along with partner Susan Jordan). Rather than enter a plea, Cumings issued a demurrer, acknowledging the charge but claiming there was no legal basis for a lawsuit.[92]

BOWLAND V. MUNICIPAL COURT: THE LIMITATIONS OF CONSTITUTIONAL PRIVACY RIGHTS

Linda Bennett remembers how she, Bowland, and Walker ended up choosing Cumings to represent them: "We liked the really straightforward Ann Flower Cumings." Other attorneys they interviewed, including Charles Garry, chief counsel to the Black Panthers in the late 1960s, proposed putting them on trial and arguing that they were not guilty because midwives had been delivering babies for centuries. "We liked the fact that she said 'we're going to appeal the fact that [you] were busted in the first place.' Which was our point of view—why the hell were we busted in the first place?"[93] They had not committed any crime. The fact that Cumings was a woman and a feminist also appealed to them, and when she told them she was also pregnant, that sealed the deal.

As Cumings got to work on the case, she realized its potential to go beyond the simple fact that the midwives had been set up and that no birth had actually taken place. This was an opportunity to make a larger claim about how the law defined and regulated birth in the United States. As the *Santa Cruz Sentinel* reported on September 1, 1974, Cumings, "citing her own pregnancy as an example, repeatedly asserted that pregnancy and childbirth are not a disease."[94] Her argument drew on the 1956 decision *Banti v. Texas*, in which a midwife was charged with practicing medicine without a license and for unlawfully treating the mother "for a disease and physical disorder." While initially convicted, the charge was overturned on appeal because the state had "not defined the practice of medicine so as to include the act of assisting women in parturition or childbirth."[95] Cumings argued there was no legal basis for the charge against the Santa Cruz midwives in municipal court in May of 1974 and again in Superior Court in September.

This line of argument proved unsuccessful. Both times, the judge denied the demurer—much to the delight of Assistant DA Bill Kelsay, who said to the judge, "it's about time somebody thinks of the rights of the (unborn) child." Proponents of the Birth Center might be able to argue that a woman should be able to do what she wants with her body, "but somebody should watch out for the child as well."[96] In the early 1970s, this would have made a powerful statement, foreshadowing many of the debates surrounding maternal/fetal rights and "personhood" issues that would intensify abortion politics in the 1980s. Implicit in Kelsay's claim is the notion that a home birth was not in the best interest of child, but rather a selfish desire on the part of pregnant women more interested in controlling their bodies than protecting their children (a claim that continues to be made by opponents of home birth). One can only imagine the reaction of the pregnant attorney and her pregnant client to these remarks in the courtroom.[97]

DA Kelsay did not explicitly make reference to abortion or *Roe v. Wade* (1973) at this point in the case, but he did make it clear that he believed politics played a role. After the arrests, he was flooded with protest letters from all over the world, according to the *San Francisco Bay Guardian*. "More women than I might wish feel an interest in the case," he explained to the *Guardian* reporter, "because they feel the doctors do abuse them." The problem, as he saw it, was that the case had taken on too much weight. "I just wish they weren't so gung-ho lib on it," he said. "I've got two lady attorneys making me feel like a male chauvinist pig."[98]

Hoping to move up the judicial ranks, Kelsay was undoubtedly reluctant to have his reputation sullied by a case that he believed had been blown out of proportion by feminist activists. His fears were most likely exacerbated by the claims of civil rights attorney Charles Garry. In the *Rolling Stone* coverage of the Santa Cruz bust, he had the last word. "Garry believes the Santa Cruz case is 'a major battle for women's liberation. The arrests were an invasion of the rights of women. The courts have no business sticking their damn noses into women's affairs. It's just plain persecution.'"[99]

Cumings initially chose not to respond to Kelsay's concerns about the rights of unborn children, continuing to focus on medicine and licensure rather than abortion politics as she appealed the decision of the Superior Court judge. In her opening brief for the appellate court in January of 1975, she reiterated her claim that birth was not a medical event and therefore midwifery was not the practice of medicine. Further, the California legislature, she argued, "has never intended to deprive a woman in pregnancy or childbirth of the assistance of any person of her choosing, whether that person was licensed or not."[100]

The question of licensure was suddenly key to the case. As of January 1, 1975—that very month—certified nurse-midwives working under physician supervision could finally practice legally in the state, a measure that had been introduced by California State Senator Anthony Beilenson. Some attributed the quick passage of the act to the Bowland case and the letters of support written at the suggestion of the Birth Center the day after the bust. Others, however, see this as unrelated, believing that the act was intended to get prenatal care to rural areas where ob/gyns were scarce. For lay midwives such as Bowland, the new law served to complicate matters. Now, their lack of licensure served to further stigmatize them, while the state recognition of certified nurse-midwives underscored the belief that midwifery was indeed the practice of medicine.[101] Thus, it became more challenging to make the claim that Bowland, Bennett, and Walker were not breaking the law because midwifery was not the practice of medicine. Cumings undoubtedly realized she needed to rethink her line of argumentation.

Before she had a chance to articulate a new strategy, one was placed in front of her, and the implications were enormous. In early 1975 the Northern California ACLU and the Santa Cruz Friends of Midwives filed an amicus brief in appellate court that placed *Roe v. Wade* front and center in the case. "Surely the principle that makes one woman's choice decisive in the abortion situation should be broad enough to protect another woman's choice as to the manner and circumstances in which her baby should be born," they wrote; "the decision to give birth is entitled to equal dignity with the decision to abort."[102] A woman's right to choose, they argued, should include all aspects of reproductive decisions, not just pregnancy termination.[103]

But the linkage to *Roe* backfired, and the state turned their argument on its head in order to weaken their case. In a respondent's brief, state attorneys labeled the claim as "glib," instead using *Roe* as evidence that the state had every right to regulate where and how babies are born. In fact, they argued, "the State has a compelling interest in the health of the mother after the first trimester, and a compelling interest in the health and welfare of potential human life after viability, thus permitting regulations reasonably related to those interests." *Roe* may have empowered women to make decisions early in pregnancy, but it empowered the state to expand its control later in pregnancy's later stages. DA Kelsay couldn't have argued it better when he praised the court for "looking out for the rights of the (unborn) child." It was right there in the *Roe* decision.[104]

Linda Bennett remembers how angry she was when *Roe* entered the debate. "That so pissed us off that we decided as a group that we were not going to promote the fact that that had happened. Because we did not want anybody else to take that as a precedent for controlling female reproduction."[105] Like it or not, Cumings knew she had to respond and that she had to distance the case from abortion politics, despite her alliances. She and her partner attorney returned to the debate surrounding the boundaries of medicine. "It must be noted," they wrote in May of 1975, "that *Roe* specifically addressed itself to the question of abortion, a stated 'medical procedure' which is clearly within the terms of 'practice of medicine'. Under no circumstances can the government argue that midwives or those persons assisting in birth do such abortions."[106] In other words, abortion might be a medical procedure, but childbirth was not. Conflation of the two was therefore problematic. If anything, a woman's right to choose where and with whom to give birth—in support of life, rather than the termination of it—should have the support of the courts as a privacy right. It was pro-natal. They had been forced into a corner, and the only way out was to divorce their cause from that of abortion rights.

The court disagreed with Cuming's defense and in December of 1976 issued its decision. Though the constitutional right to privacy had been "substantially expanded to protect certain personal choices pertaining to child-rearing, marriage, and procreation," it has "never been interpreted so broadly as to protect a woman's choice of the manner and circumstances in which her baby is born"—indeed, the "state's interest in the life of the unborn child supersedes the woman's own privacy right." Thus, in this context, *Roe* became a vehicle to constrain reproductive rights, rather than expand them.

Cumings was furious with the decision and promptly submitted a petition for rehearing. This time, however, she centered her argument on the less contentious idea of a "zone of privacy" articulated in cases such as *Griswold v. Connecticut* (1965) and *Eisenstadt v. Baird* (1972), both centered on the right of individuals to use contraception. American adults had been granted the right to sexual privacy by the court—and that should, she argued, include the act of giving birth. "The mother is entitled to the privacy that the birthing process demands," wrote Cumings. "Giving birth is a sexual act. She has the right to consummate her sexual activity with consenting adults in the privacy of her home. Her relationship with her midwife is a personal,

sexual relationship, conducted in private."[107] Rather than engage with what
she probably viewed as a hopeless case (attempting to extend reproductive
right of privacy beyond abortion), she deflected it, drawing instead on the
claims of Lang and Bowland, along with transpersonal psychologists such
as Stan Grof, that birth was a sexual act. If the right to abortion was controversial, the right to sexual privacy was certainly less so.

But the request was denied, and the decision stood. *Bowland v. Municipal
Court* would later be cited in many other cases to justify the state regulation and restriction of midwifery practice in order to allegedly protect the
interests of the unborn.[108] Opponents of home birth undoubtedly realized that the most effective way of discouraging the practice was to clamp
down on those providing the service, rather than to question the privacy
rights of a laboring mother.[109] If no midwives were able to legally assist at
home birth, then women were more likely to deliver in a hospital, they rea-
soned.[110] Thus the focus on practitioner rather than patient (at least in the
courts) continued to rise, and self-proclaimed midwives increasingly found
themselves under heightened legal scrutiny.

Cumings' decision to distance childbirth from abortion in her legal argument may also have been motivated by local politics. In March of 1975,
the state had forced the Santa Cruz Women's Health Collective (unrelated
to the SCBC) to close its health clinic, ostensibly because they lacked sufficient medical backup in case of any complication from abortion. But the
Collective believed something else was the cause, as they were following
similar procedures as in other California counties. "Compared to other CA
counties, Santa Cruz is one of the most backward and conservative in relation to abortion care." They reported experiencing "antagonism" and "hostility" from the medical community and believed it stemmed from the fact
that they were a group of "non-professionals working collectively to challenge the type of health care women usually get and to provide an alternative to that."[111] This was, of course, exactly what the Santa Cruz midwives
were doing. But the different context—pregnancy termination versus
birth—prevented a successful alliance between the two groups. It also
underscored the limitations of the *Roe* decision, particularly its inability to
bring an increasingly fractured cohort of activists under the larger umbrella
of reproductive rights, even if many of its members identified with multiple
aspects of the campaign.[112]

THE END OF THE SANTA CRUZ BIRTH CENTER

By the time of the State Supreme Court decision, the Santa Cruz Birth
Center had already disbanded. In part, this stemmed from the center's

growing popularity as media coverage and the Birth Center Defense Committee kept the bust in the spotlight. Bowland later recalled that "at the time, the media was really supportive. We had very good press.... There wasn't a lot of negative publicity."[113] Such attention, however, would soon overwhelm the center. Women came from all over to train with the famous "outlaws." Sharon Steiner came from the Emma Goldman women's health clinic in Iowa City to train at the Santa Cruz Birth Center, with the intention of starting a birth center back in Iowa. "This is the place where it all began, you know," she explained. But she was disappointed with the haphazard method of training in Santa Cruz. "One of the things I wanted to do was to come here and learn from somebody who's already experienced. Kind of an apprentice relationship, and that just hasn't worked out at all," she explained. "You go to a birth as the third person, take notes, and after 5–10 of these, you start assisting. Then you become a co-midwife." Birth Center midwives were overwhelmed with the Bowland case, running the center, and tending to births, and "no one had energy left over for training people and they would get burned out and leave," she explained. "I'm still getting over my disappointment."[114]

Another Birth Center midwife described a breakdown in communication. "People were playing less and less attention to each other because once the workload got so heavy the interaction between us became—that was the thing that was dropped . . . the emphasis we need to put into the community is education."[115] It was not until the creation of the Seattle Midwifery School a few years later that lay midwives began to seriously grapple with the issue of formal education.

By 1975, none of the founders of the Birth Center remained; seven others had taken their place. But it was not just the practitioners who changed; so had the clientele. Midwifery was "no longer the favor among friends as it was," Karen Ehrlich explained.[116] "The people at the beginning who came to the birth center were people who were pretty much prepared to have birth at home alone whether or not someone was there," recalled Kristin Thomas, who trained there in 1975. They were happy to have the help, but they would have done it anyway. By 1975, however, people were coming "because we are there—not because they are capable of doing it themselves." Sharon Hamilton, who came from Florida to work with the midwives in the mid-1970s, agreed. "One of the hassles that has developed is that people come wanting to place responsibility on our shoulders rather than wanting to take responsibility for themselves."[117] Something had been lost in the process.

Nonetheless, the symbol of the Santa Cruz Birth Center remained potent. The fact that it had survived as long as it had was significant, an indicator of northern California's openness to alternative birth. "A lot of the reason why this is happening here is because this community is such that it can happen here," explained one midwife, "even though there are things blocking our way, it's not half so—it's not so much of a struggle as it would be in other places."[118] At the epicenter of the counterculture, it wasn't surprising that Santa Cruz would attract a large number of young people interested in home birth. Kate Bowland described what was happening by the mid-1970s as "isolated pockets of consciousness" cropping up in particular places.[119] Santa Cruz was among the first.

Within midwifery circles, the Birth Center bust represented the power of organized medicine to quash alternative birth. Among feminists, it suggested the limitations of reproductive rights arguments and the law. To the extent that the case has been analyzed by scholars, the focus has been on the 1976 decision and the use of *Roe* to prevent direct-entry midwives from obtaining licensure or being recognized by the state.[120] But the story behind the creation of the Santa Cruz Birth Center was far richer than a legal lens alone can capture. Lang, Bennett, and Bowland brought curiosity, determination, art, politics, and medicine into the teepees and bedrooms of laboring women. They collaborated with (and sometimes challenged) doctors, organized seminars and defense committees, taught birth classes, trained other midwives, published books, wrote poetry, and read the *Communist Manifesto* alongside Grof's theories of rebirthing and *Gray's Anatomy*. They had the wherewithal to capitalize on the publicity from the bust and to portray themselves as outlaws, so that their case would not be forgotten. They forced the state to rethink—and eventually change—outdated statutes regarding midwifery. And they helped discover and define what they believed to be a new profession, blending art, psychology, science, and even collaborative medicine with the ancient practice of midwifery.

CHAPTER 5

୶

From El Paso to Lexington

The Formation of the Midwives Alliance
of North America

O n May 5, 2012—International Midwives' Day—the Midwives Alliance of North America (MANA) launched a public education campaign on YouTube. "I am a Midwife" profiled a number of midwives across the country in short interviews, in order to put faces to the title. "People don't tend to know what's a midwife," explained MANA president Geradine Simkins. The introductory "Sneak Peek!" included white, Latina, African American, and Native American women speaking with pride and passion about their profession. Being a midwife, explained Claudia Booker, "brings you to the door of revolution." Living in Washington, D.C., "a city where the basic color is shades of black," she is "committed to serving people of color."[1] So is Marinah Farrell, who became the first woman of color to serve as MANA president in 2014. She grew up "in a place between the Mexican and U.S. borders" and believes in working for "vulnerable populations" because her parents were both involved in missionary work.[2] For her, being a midwife means "love and compassion, good care, safety, freedom, feminism, and social justice."[3] Over 26,000 YouTube viewers have heard Booker and Farrell describe what the profession of midwifery means to them.

The "I am a Midwife" campaign marks one of MANA's most recent efforts to package midwifery as a meaningful, compassionate, and revolutionary profession. It is an important step toward recognizing disparities in maternity care as well as honoring diversity within the profession. But the goal of putting a face to the name "midwife" dates back to the roots of MANA's formation decades ago.

WHO IS A MIDWIFE?

In the lobby of the historic Paso del Norte Hotel in El Paso, Texas, a two-story banner greeted the 250 or so registrants who had traveled from forty-one states and four countries for one January weekend in 1977. "WELCOME first international conference of practicing midwives," the sign proclaimed. Mahogany woodwork, black serpentine marble, and an elaborate Tiffany glass dome surrounded the participants who arrived via buses, vans, and airplanes to the most formal, organized affair that lay midwives practicing in the United States had ever seen.[4]

This meeting was truly something new. A reporter from *Mothering* magazine sent to cover the conference noted that she didn't even know how to pronounce "midwifery" when she received her assignment. Walking into the lobby of the grand hotel, she saw for the first time the disparate group of women who embraced the ancient term and declared it alive and well. "If someone were to ask me what a typical midwife looked like, I wouldn't be able to tell them," the reporter wrote. "Some looked like nurses, having that air of professionalism about them. Some were outgoing and some were more reserved. Some were young and some were old. . . . Some were dressed in suits, but most were dressed in 'hippie' style clothing. I could not point to any one person and say, 'there is a midwife.'"[5]

Carol Leonard ransacked all of her favorite New Hampshire thrift stores in search of her conference attire, choosing a 1940s gray flannel suit and a black beret with a silk rose attached to make her initial appearance.[6] Though she was no stranger to midwifery, she was struck by the colorful assortment of characters. "I really feel like a country mouse as I stand in the ornate lobby of the Grand Hotel, clutching my brocade suitcase. What culture shock. There are midwives everywhere, all different shapes and sizes! There are sleek, cosmopolitan nurse-midwives from medical centers; groups of colorfully dressed Mexican parteras, chattering excitedly in Spanish; and many apprentice-trained midwives, like me."[7]

The conference was not limited to lay midwives; reporters, representatives from consumer groups, childbirth educators, videographers, and a handful of doctors and certified nurse-midwives also attended, providing support, information, documentation, and ideas about how to promote midwifery and home birth. "There were babies everywhere, all ages, and all nursing," and a laboring mother awaited checkups from her midwife (who also happened to be one of the conference organizers, Shari Daniels) in a hotel room upstairs.[8]

Photographs and written descriptions convey the singularity of the moment, as participants first laid eyes on underground midwives they had only read about. "It was inspiring to finally meet all these women who through their writings have represented the plight of midwives for so many years," recalled midwife and co-organizer Fran Ventre. This was a group that for the first several years of its existence had remained for the most part intentionally invisible, hoping not to draw attention to its questionable professional and legal status. Now, for a brief moment, midwives shared a physical space, a platform, an agenda, and several goals. "To describe the First International Conference of Practicing Midwives is almost impossible," Ventre stated. "How can one capture in words the spirit, emotions and feelings of bonding that happened to all of us dedicated to bringing the art of midwifery back to childbirth?"[9]

Yet many did attempt to describe what was gained in the three-day gathering. They sensed that this was history in the making and wanted to help record it. They also hoped that their voices and stories would redefine American midwifery as a movement far more radical than that characterized by certified nurse-midwives. Ideologically, many of them viewed midwifery as a feminist endeavor that enabled women to reclaim their bodies, rather than being controlled by the medical profession. Barred from membership in the American College of Nurse Midwives, they sought to create a more inclusive organization that could provide them with the protection, legitimacy, and visibility needed to sustain and grow their trade. This would turn out to be an enormously challenging task.

The conference program included a wide range of presentations and workshops, starting on Friday evening with an introductory session of seasoned veterans. All the big players were there, which added to the sense that something major was taking place. Most of the participants would have been familiar with the names of the women who shared the podium that night, many feeling "star-struck" as they listened to Ina May Gaskin, Raven Lang, Suzanne Arms, Fran Ventre, and Ann Flower Cumings.[10] "Many of my heroes are here," proclaimed Carol Leonard, "the women who are the foundation stones of this new movement. They are charismatic, skilled, feisty, articulate, opinionated, wild, and beautiful midwives."[11]

These featured speakers were the trailblazers, the ones who had already made history. They viewed lay midwifery as inherently political, influenced by other social movements including civil rights, anti-war, feminism, and consumer rights. They believed that what gave lay midwifery power and legitimacy was its connection to these other movements. It was time to tell their story. "If you remain true to the battle to get out the truth, the movement will grow, expand and have power," stated feminist attorney Ann Flower Cumings. "Movements have made it past legal barriers before and history teaches us that they will again."[12] Legalizing lay midwifery was therefore the natural next step.

Cumings was joined by other birth luminaries. Ina May Gaskin traveled from The Farm along with husband Stephen Gaskin, midwife assistant Margaret Nofziger, a film crew, and two Guatemalan midwives. She spoke of the 570 births that Farm midwives had attended since 1970, only nineteen of which took place in a hospital. Co-organizer Fran Ventre came from the Washington, D.C. area, where she ran Home Oriented Maternity Experience (H.O.M.E.). Raven Lang and Suzanne Arms' names and faces were perhaps the best known of the group. Raven had started the Santa Cruz Birth Center and published the *Birth Book*, which was featured in Suzanne Arms' bestselling expose, *Immaculate Deception*. "That's like seeing Elvis," remarked Ventre on her first encounter with Raven Lang.[13] Together, these speakers set a fiery tone for the next two days and articulated the lofty goals of the conference: to bring midwives together, to share resources, and to create a national association.

El Paso was a powerful moment of convergence. "The room was full of weeping women," Santa Cruz midwife Karen Ehrlich remembered, her eyes glistening. "I remember the feeling of solidarity of having people from all over the place coming together for the very first time, talking to each other, sharing experiences, learning new things from each other, connecting in a heart space that there was no other place, anywhere, where any of us had had that kind of experience of coming together." The meeting was something that, decades later, she could still recall in great detail. "It was incredible . . . Earth-shattering . . . Something I will never forget."[14]

But it was also a moment of dissonance, as participants struggled to articulate and agree upon goals and priorities. It was one thing to recognize their common bond as underground midwives; it was quite another to channel that sense of solidarity into creating an actual organization. From the very beginning, four major issues—public image, cost, leadership, and training—threatened to undermine that goal.

Ideas expressed at the El Paso meeting reflected larger trends in American culture with regard to medicine. Beginning in the mid-1960s, surveys indicated a drastic loss of confidence in organized medicine, as well as a rise in the number of Americans who believed they had suffered from a negative medical care experience.[15] Consumers began seeking new, often alternative sources of medical advice and treatment. Acupuncture, herbal remedies, and homeopathy, along with home birth, became increasingly acceptable. These practices were brought into wider circulation by a boom in health publishing.[16] Raven Lang's *Birth Book*, Suzanne Arms' *Immaculate*

Deception, and Ina May Gaskin's *Spiritual Midwifery*, among many others, inspired readers to question hospital policies on childbirth and to consider giving birth at home under the care of a lay midwife. Conference organizers were galvanized not only by these books and the rising interest in home birth, but also by the larger consumer movement to challenge mainstream medical practices. A close investigation of the dynamics leading up to this meeting, as well as the one held in Lexington five years later, reveals how midwives and consumers were able to create a professional organization open to all midwives and their supporters by the early 1980s.

EL PASO: ROOTS, CHALLENGES, AND GOALS

The three midwives who organized the El Paso conference (Fran Ventre, Shari Daniels, and Nancy Mills) first met a year earlier, at the first annual conference of the National Association of Parents and Professionals for Safe Alternatives in Childbirth (NAPSAC) in Washington, D.C.[17] NAPSAC was a consumer nonprofit founded in 1975 by David and Lee Stewart, a married couple whose five children were all born at home, some without an attendant. Frustrated by the lack of programs, education, or practitioners supportive of home birth in their home state of Missouri, the Stewarts vowed to promote home birth as a safe alternative to hospital birth.

NAPSAC was just one of many consumer organizations formed in the 1970s as part of a powerful grassroots movement demanding better health care. Groups such as Public Citizen's Health Research Group and the National Women's Health Network fostered the "consumerist concept of patient as watchdog."[18] Reports exposing disturbing cases of patient experimentation and questionable ethics, such as the Tuskegee Syphilis Study, galvanized interest in forming consumer groups to monitor and challenge patient treatment.[19] In terms of childbirth reform, a large number of middle-class white parents interested in reclaiming their rights as parents mobilized to make their own decisions about pregnancy, childbirth, and childrearing.

According to La Leche League president Marian Tompson, there were about 650 people in attendance from all over the United States at the 1976 NAPSAC conference in Washington, D.C., "representing all types of people." It seemed to her that the majority was "middle class and straight."[20] About half of the participants were members of La Leche League, underscoring the important connections between maternity care and breastfeeding. There were also certified nurse-midwives, lay midwives, and physicians at the meeting. If she was accurate in her demographic assessment, this would reflect what had become a trend in patients' and consumer rights groups. What had started as a movement to improve health care services for the "minority poor" resulted in a recognition that the white middle class was also deprived of rightful treatment.[21] Attendance at the NAPSAC conference suggested the extent to which consumer groups supportive of home birth appeared to be directed at the white middle class.

The NAPSAC conference inspired many of the attending midwives to offer a similar type of meeting for midwives. Consumer interest in home birth thus played a significant role in the organization of lay midwives. As Ventre recalls, "we got together and somehow we started talking about the need for a separate conference just for midwives. We decided that the three of us would try to do this together."[22] According to Ventre, Shari Daniels, who ran the Maternity Center at El Paso, agreed to sponsor the conference and did most of the organizational work. Nancy Mills, a lay midwife working in northern California and featured in *Immaculate Deception*, was in charge of West Coast recruiting, advertising, and organizing speakers, while Ventre took care of the East Coast.

As the three began planning, they quickly encountered four basic organizational questions. First, what sort of public image did they want to promote? As with the creators of the 2012 "I am a Midwife" campaign, these organizers recognized the importance of putting a face to the name in order to gain visibility and recognition from the wider community. Second, given the limited economic resources of lay midwives, how could they make the conference both professional and affordable? Third, who should be chosen as speakers to represent lay midwives? And fourth, what sort of training should be required in order to gain expertise? These issues, which first emerged during the planning stages, continue to challenge the midwifery community.

Ventre tackled the image issue. Since she had experience with the layout and design of her organization's newsletter, *News from H.O.M.E.*, she volunteered to take care of the conference program, including creating the cover. She asked the graphic artist who had drawn sketches for her newsletter, Carolyne Landon, to design a logo. Landon worked as a courtroom artist for NBC television and the *Washington Post* but was also a home birth client of Ventre who lived on the Zany Ramorski Farm, a health care commune run by physician and comedian Patch Adams. Ventre delivered Landon's child on the farm, accepting Landon's artistic services as payment in lieu of cash payment.

Landon's first work was a sketch of a traditional nineteenth-century midwife, to accompany Ventre's article on how she got licensed as a lay midwife in Maryland. This was a surprising choice, because Ventre sometimes intentionally distanced herself from earlier midwives, who had been denigrated by public health campaigns and organized medicine as uneducated and unsanitary. "Contrary to the stereotype, we [lay midwives] are not a modern day version of the old crone of midwife folklore, unkempt and illiterate," she announced at a conference of certified nurse-midwives in 1976.[23]

Landon's second illustration accompanied a H.O.M.E. newsletter cover story on current licensure status in different states. This time, Landon sketched her image of a modern midwife—wearing bellbottoms, Birkenstock sandals, hoop earrings, a kerchief over her hair, and a hippie shoulder bag—modeled on Ventre herself.

For the conference logo, Landon created a composite portrait of the two sketches, "with the older 'granny' being in half tones like a spiritual being behind the modern midwife walking in sync."[24] The dress, hair, and instrument bag had been updated, but the faces were identical, both bearing a look of determination and commitment. This was a powerful and

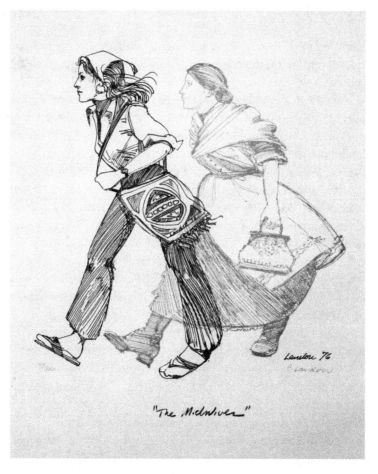

Figure 5.1 Conference logo designed by Carolyne Landon. Wendy Kline personal collection. Reprinted with permission by Carolyne Landon.

provocative image that portrayed the lay midwife, rather than the certified nurse-midwife, as the central figure of the movement. It suggested that she would carry the torch of midwifery care. By juxtaposing the two images, Landon was also connecting the 1970s lay midwife with earlier generations of midwives.

Midwife Shari Daniels dealt with the financial matters and local arrangements. She chose her home town of El Paso and the Paso del Norte Hotel. She set registration fees at $55, with meals costing another $30, a steep price for many lay midwives who could barely make ends meet. Yet many still desperately wanted to come when they learned about the conference.

Subscribers to Ventre's H.O.M.E. newsletter (there were about 2,000 in 1976) learned that one goal of the conference was to establish a national association to offer support and guidance to midwives across the United States. On the last day the group would elect representatives, form an organization, and establish a newsletter "to facilitate nation-wide communication among midwives."[25] These lofty goals motivated many to have their interests represented at the conference. They believed that it was time for all midwives to have a national organization.

The issue of who would be invited to speak at such an important meeting generated controversy. When word got out that doctors had been invited as keynote speakers, some protested. "We question the validity of institutionally trained medical personnel in a primary teaching capacity at this conference," wrote twelve midwives working at Birthcenter in California. Had the conference organizers completely forgotten what these lay midwives were fighting against? "Midwifery is not pathological obstetrics!" Lay midwives were demanding a radical break from obstetrical birth. "The very nature of our training is in the home, not the institutions, and lay midwifery is not so much about obstetrics as about women controlling their own lives," they asserted.[26] This was a feminist issue. The politics surrounding the place of birth—and who held the power—needed to be reflected in the slate of conference speakers.

Not only were these speakers doctors, but they were men. Women's health activists had argued since the beginning of the decade that women could not achieve full equality without the right to reclaim their bodies. Doctors were overwhelmingly male (in 1970, only 7.6 percent of physicians and 7.2 percent of obstetrician-gynecologists were female), and, according to critics, paternalistic, condescending, and judgmental.[27]

When Santa Cruz midwife Allee Jay received a copy of the conference brochure in the mail, she was disturbed to discover the number of male doctors speaking. "Can men really know about birth or midwifery on a gut level?" she asked organizer Shari Daniels. All of the male speakers, she pointed out, had the word "problem" in their paper titles, which to her indicated their assumption that birth was a pathological process. Dr. Don Creevy, an obstetrician at Stanford University Hospital, was due to speak on "The Importance of Recognizing Problems" in pre- and postnatal care; naturopathic and chiropractic physician N. B. Ettinghausen on "Problems in Labor and Delivery"; obstetrician Tom Brewer on "Problems of Poor Nutrition"; and pediatrician Michael Witte on "Newborn Examination, Problems of the Newborn, and Newborn Resuscitation."[28]

She drafted a letter of complaint that she shared with her midwifery study group, which met regularly in the San Francisco Bay area. "There was general agreement that it spoke for many of us," one member wrote.[29] Most of them knew these doctors and were familiar with their arguments. Jay made a bold proposal: "why not have midwives from the West Coast head the seminars in place of the scheduled male speakers?" They could reiterate some of the doctors' points, but in their own words. "Let's at least challenge the status quo and not take a back seat to professionals," she suggested.[30].

Daniels, though sympathetic, felt the need to provide conference participants with training from experts. "Could I begin by saying that we identify with your feelings and agree with so many of your comments that your letter could be an echo of one of our conversations around here!" exclaimed Daniels. But she disagreed with Jay's desire to see an "emphasis placed on <u>normalcy</u>, and on <u>midwives</u> sharing amongst ourselves."[31]

Was the goal of this conference to educate and protect the reputation of lay midwives at a time when no formal training, certification, or standards were in place? Or was it an opportunity to empower and legitimize an underground grassroots network of women who viewed their work as primarily political rather than medical? The first goal required the presence of outside experts, while the second refuted them.

Daniels began to realize it could not do both. "Many suggestions were received and we really do feel that this will be a unique chance for all midwives to come together in one place for the first time," she explained. Based on the enthusiastic descriptions of the conference, clearly she met that goal—at least for those who could afford to attend.

Then Daniels explained her reason for prioritizing training over accessibility. "I believe myself from the hundreds of letters we have received from across the country that the primary need expressed over and over again by midwives all across the country was for training in those aspects of midwifery that are simply not covered in the hit-or-miss type of apprentice training most of them have had." Many physicians remained hostile to lay midwives, but the ones selected to speak at the conference were enthusiastic supporters of the cause.

It was a valuable opportunity to demonstrate publicly the potential for building alliances with at least a small part of the established medical profession. "Remember that there are only two or three places in the entire country where midwives have had the advantage of give-and-take working relationships with any type of physician. Most midwives have no access at all to this type of detailed, rather specialized knowledge about how to handle problems that may arise and they feel a deep insecurity knowing their ignorance. Not ALL births are ideal." Thus, the conference would provide the knowledge and the skills that could empower and protect midwives in all circumstances, not just the good outcomes.

Daniels still believed that the other organizational goals—creating a powerful public image and developing leadership—were important. "Midwives DO need to come together, to share, to develop their own specific midwifery skills, to write new textbooks—amen and amen to all of those ideas and we couldn't agree with you more." Future organization was essential. "We need to start planning such professional meetings immediately, along with correspondence courses, professional newsletters/ journals, books, and you name it—maybe meeting on a regional basis that would enable more midwives to come with little expense."

Here, she finally made reference to the financial issue, acknowledging that not everyone would be able to afford to come to El Paso, but suggesting that there would be future opportunities. Courses, newsletters, and regional meetings would enable midwives who were too distant, too poor, or too busy to come to a national meeting, to still play an important part in the development of a professional identity. This could happen in the future. "But this first meeting was primarily to meet the expressed need of so many of us who NEED the knowledge we have been prevented from acquiring—and to enable us to get together for the first time to decide where we go from here. We can't do everything the first weekend we get together!"[32]

Yet many did not think these were the right priorities if so many midwives could not afford to participate. "Once again we get left out because we're poor," wrote the twelve Birthcenter midwives. "The required fees are affordable only to professional persons and organizations, and are blatantly unreasonable to lay persons." They demanded that their letter serve as their registration. "Travel fees and time away from our Birthcenter is the most we can spend," they declared. But it was essential that they attend, claiming "our input is vital." [33]

Santa Cruz midwife Allee Jay also could not afford the cost of registration. "I, like many local midwives, make little money doing births. Some of us are in school and doing few births. I personally have an income of $190 a month to support me and my son; I can't afford the price of the conference. I know of approximately 30 other midwives in the Santa

Cruz, Monterrey, San Jose and San Francisco Bay areas who can't afford the fee either."

Jay pleaded with the conference organizers to grant at least some of the Santa Cruz midwives scholarships. "Our community's midwives who were part of the former Santa Cruz Birth Center, to whom countless women have come for information and training, should be well represented," she argued. "Without scholarships we will probably be unable to attend." [34] Organizer Fran Ventre agreed. "In retrospect," she wrote Jay apologetically, "the fees for the conference are steep (considering the fact that lay midwives usually don't charge severe prices for their services and aren't $$ oriented)."[35] She felt strongly that the Santa Cruz midwives should attend, in part because they had played such a crucial role in birth politics in the early 1970s.

Daniels disagreed. Not all midwives needed to attend the conference. Since the conference would be audio and videotaped, and booths would display the most recent books and articles on the subject, anyone could convey the conference content to their hometown. "That is exactly what we have suggested to others who are facing your problem," she wrote to Jay. "Send your best qualified and most experienced person and plan to have training sessions afterward for everyone else to share the material. We can only accommodate 400–500 attendants at the conference and we know ourselves that this number is too limited to meet the need of all those who want to come, even if there were no problems of financing to deal with."[36]

Exchanges between conference organizers and discontented lay midwives reveal conflicting visions of what should happen at the first national conference of midwives and who should represent the group. Letter writers felt that their presence was crucial—not because of a need for training or information (as suggested by Daniels), but for representation. "We want to voice our views on liscensing [sic], on training programs, on competence standards, based on our own unique and valid experiences," wrote the twelve Birthcenter midwives. "Although we can agree with the stated goals, there are no provisions for us to have input into the decision making structure. The elections are meant to be the way, yet these seem much like a popularity contest." This was exacerbated by the fact that all nominations for representatives would be drawn from those physically present at the conference. "The logical way to form a national organization would be to hold a planning workshop at the conference," they argued. "This would accurately reflect the needs and concerns of practicing lay midwives who are seriously interested in forming this organization. What you have done is present the organization already structured without input from the people who are expected to support, fund, and participate in it."[37]

While none of these twelve midwives would end up attending the conference, the concerns they articulated would become major challenges for midwives over the next few decades. If midwifery was an art, rather than a science, why should it be regulated? Would certification and licensure turn midwives into mini-doctors, and thus contributors to a system they were fighting against? As lay midwife (and conference organizer) Nancy Mills asked during the conference, "Do we want to be obstetricians? And if we want to be obstetricians, let's go to medical school. If we want to be midwives in the true sense of the *natural practitioner*, let's try to remain natural and really be able to keep our feet on the ground and protect that place."[38]

Sociologist Raymond DeVries articulated this as the "dilemma of licensure," citing a 1977 home birth study on the effects of licensing. "A license isn't really a guarantee of expertise: Anyone graduated from medical school can legally deliver babies, even if they've had the experience of only three or four deliveries." Yet unlicensed midwives with much more experience were legally barred. "Medical licensing diminishes any accountability to people, the 'consumer', in favor of accountability to a licensing board."[39] DeVries concluded in 1985 that "state sanction to practice does not bring autonomy to midwives, but rather formalizes the dominance of physicians over them."[40]

Though many midwives disagreed, believing that licensure was a necessary step toward self-sufficiency, the majority at the conference felt that it was not the right time and not under the right leadership. Gaskin remembers that "there was an attempt to organize a midwifes' organization at the time, but I wasn't comfortable with the way it was coming down." She echoed the concerns of the twelve Birthcenter midwives who had written Daniels. "It appeared to me that it was going to be some kind of hierarchical deal, and I didn't feel I wanted to be much of a part of that. I was a little worried about the prematurity of it and the way it was happening."

Gaskin did, however, support the idea of creating a national newsletter and volunteered her printing press at The Farm to produce it. "The Practicing Midwife" later became the *Birth Gazette*, published by The Farm until 2000. The El Paso conference, according to Gaskin, was "kickoff time. It was out of the conference that the discussion came of the need for midwives to open lines of communication." [41] Lay midwife publications such as *The Practicing Midwife* would enable such communication to occur more effectively than at a weekend conference.

Although the organizers had saved Sunday afternoon to announce the newly elected representatives to a national organization, no such election occurred. "A NATIONAL MIDWIFERY ASSOCIATION AT LAST," they announced in the conference program, but it was nothing more than wishful thinking for the time being. Too many agreed with Ina May Gaskin that such a move would threaten their livelihood.

Instead, someone suggested devoting Sunday afternoon to an "open mic" session. "This turned out to be the highlight of the entire conference," wrote a reporter for *Mothering*.[42] Though Daniels was initially dead set against having anyone speak at the conference who wasn't on the program, she relented after heated lobbying, as many midwives wanted the opportunity to voice their opinions. No one felt ready to concede to Daniels. Choosing the most effective, qualified representatives and leaders required forethought and discussion.

Participants weighed in on everything from organizational strategies to birth experiences to future directions. "It was an incredible outpouring of all the different philosophies and persuasions that the rebirth of midwifery was based in," Karen Ehrlich remembers. "As woman after woman got up to speak her mind and heart, we experienced elation, anger, frustration, humor, delight, bonding, exhilaration and many many tears."[43] They concluded by joining hands in a giant circle around the conference hall to sing a ballad written by one of the Santa Cruz midwives, "The Daughters of Time."[44] Ventre reported that "there was much love generated as our voices blended together in the spiritual OM."

Despite differences in opinion regarding organizational strategies, most left the conference heartened. "I [came] home, inspired with even more passion, buoyed and supported by the underground network of the wild and brave women who attend births around the country," reflected Carol Leonard.[45] "We left the conference different than when we came," wrote another participant, "charged, encouraged, enlightened, entwined in believing in ourselves and our shared purpose. As I was leaving the elevator operator wistfully confided, 'We sure are going to miss y'all'. Me too, sister, me too."[46] One imagines that even the hotel employees would never think about birth the same way again.

Six months after the El Paso conference, Warren Pearse, the Executive Director of the American College of Obstetricians and Gynecology (ACOG), issued his concern about the "anti-intellectual–anti-science revolt" against hospital birth.[47] One wonders the extent to which his statement was a direct response to the First International Conference of Practicing Midwives. Something different was afoot in the 1970s when it came to birth. Midwife and activist Rahima Baldwin labeled it the "new homebirth," marked by "women's desire to assume active responsibility for their bodies, their lives and their birth experiences."[48] While it didn't begin in El Paso, the conference was the first time that proponents of midwifery and home birth had the opportunity to meet face to face, to discover kindred spirits, and to brainstorm on how to move forward. As Fran Ventre explained, "It was the most exciting conference I can ever remember because it was the first one. We all came together and felt like, 'God, there are other nuts just like us. We're not crazy, we're not crazy."[49] El Paso would inspire more reflection and writing by a group of women well aware that they were making history and that such history should be documented. Just as they recorded the details of each labor and birth, they chronicled the painful yet exuberant process of birthing a profession, of hammering out the procedures, the methods (or non-methods), and politics that they believed would bring birth back home.

TAKING SIDES: ACNM POSITION STATEMENTS

ACOG was not the only medical association concerned about the increasing number of lay midwives cropping up in the 1970s. The American College of Nurse Midwives, formed in 1955, also struggled with how to respond. Many members expressed concern that there were perhaps thousands of women involved in delivering babies at home and calling themselves "midwives" with no formal credentials. They were also concerned about the rising consumer interest in out-of-hospital birth. Many of these consumers preferred lay midwives to CNMs, whom they viewed as being complicit with obstetricians in promoting a medical model of birth.[50] In essence, this meant that three different groups—obstetricians, certified nurse-midwives, and lay midwives—were competing for clients.

This competition forced ACNM to position itself in relation to the lay midwifery community, as well as in relation to ACOG. ACOG had only formally recognized nurse-midwifery as a legitimate branch of maternity care in 1971. The emergence of a more radical, anti-establishment group of midwives could potentially undermine ACNM's alliance with ACOG, especially given that many obstetricians did not understand the difference between a certified nurse-midwife and a lay midwife. Confusion between the two, nurse-midwives worried, "would destroy the hard and slowly won record and growing reputation of nurse-midwifery."[51]

For ACNM, two issues were at stake: the credentials of the midwife and the location of birth. Only 8% of certified nurse-midwives practicing in 1976/ early 1977 were involved in home births.[52] Like obstetricians, they voiced concern over the safety of home birth, regardless of the type of practitioner. Therefore, ACNM's initial strategy was to create a position statement on home birth—rather than a direct attack on lay midwives.

Concern about the impact of lay midwifery on the status of CNMs emerged early in the 1970s. At the ACNM executive board meeting on October 27, 1973, board member Irene Matousek "presented a problem that ACNM members in California are having," referring to the presence of the Santa Cruz Birth Center and the dramatic rise in home births across the state. According to meeting minutes, she argued that "the public associates nurse-midwifery with home delivery services and this has posed an urgent problem." In addition, another board member noted that she had been contacted by a group requesting policy recommendations for midwives interested in home deliveries. "Concern was expressed that the ACNM not be associated with home delivery services," the board determined, "which are outside of recognized health care systems." [53]

In response, the board immediately adopted and published an official position statement on home deliveries. "ACNM considers the hospital or officially approved maternity home as the site for childbirth because of the distinct advantage to the welfare of mother and child." Only these two settings could combine a "family-centered atmosphere" with the "readily available obstetric team including the physician." [54] This statement allied ACNM with ACOG's position against home birth. It also angered some ACNM members, who were not consulted in the wording or publishing of such a statement, suggesting the group was far from unified in its stance on home birth.[55] As a result the ACNM instituted new mechanisms for reviewing or initiating clinical practice statements.

As internal debate continued to circulate regarding creating an official position statement on home birth, ACNM began to focus more specifically on the increasing number of non-nurse midwives. Trying to come up with a unified statement on home birth was tricky enough. But attempting to position the organization between organized obstetrics/ACOG and anti-establishment lay midwives was even more of a political hot potato.

Certain high-ranking ACNM members recognized and articulated the difficult position nurse-midwives were in. ACNM Board member and regional representative Susan Leibel, who would play a formative role in the creation of MANA, attempted to explain this to her 202 dues-paying members in 1977. "As recognized members of the obstetric health care delivery system, we now find ourselves in the midst of a dichotomy. At one end of the spectrum the specialties of fetal–maternal medicine and neonatology with their highly developed technologies increasingly impinge on the process of 'normal' childbirth," she acknowledged. "At the other end of the spectrum, a social renaissance of 'rugged individualism' or in some cases downright fear and disgust has propelled a growing, serious movement placing limited or no reliance on health care systems for childbirth care." Where did that leave CNMs, attempting to integrate themselves more fully into established obstetrical care? "We are striving to reap the benefits of technology when it is truly needed and we are reaching out to develop acceptable quality alternatives which minimize intervention. This is no small task," she acknowledged with some concern. If forced to choose sides, with whom should they ally themselves? "At worst, the heat of the issues will burn and divide us," she warned.[56]

Leibel knew what it was like to be forced to choose sides. After becoming a nurse, she attended one of the country's few accredited nurse-midwifery programs at Columbia University, and became certified as a nurse-midwife in 1972. Leibel then moved to California, only to discover that she could not legally practice in the state, which had stopped issuing licenses to midwives in 1948. She got to know the lay midwives and activists involved in the "home birth scene," including Raven Lang, Kate Bowland, and Suzanne Arms. "I resisted involvement with the homebirth movement, and avoided contact with 'lay midwives'," she wrote to a fellow CNM in 1977.[57] Too much was at stake to ally herself with this more radical group.

In a different context, however, Leibel claimed that she "began to really respect what they were doing." She appreciated the politics of lay midwifery. "Initially I was sort of a conservative East Coast person and didn't think this was appropriate, but I really put on a more objective, critical head and said, 'Yes, they're meeting a need.'" There was clearly a growing number of consumers who for political reasons would opt for a lay midwife over any other type of practitioner. Upon reflection, she explained, "I think I began to see this as a feminist and a public health issue. I certainly have no attachment to nursing, so from that standpoint I could see midwifery as discrete. . . . So I became a supporter of direct entry midwifery."[58] She, along with a few other CNMs familiar with the lay midwives, would play a crucial role in the establishment of a new national organization.

In 1977, the ACNM created an Interorganizational Committee to track the movement of lay midwifery in the United States. As part of this task, the committee asked regional representatives to survey their members regarding their knowledge and attitudes toward lay midwifery and its relationship to nurse-midwifery. "The board recognizes that there is a diversity of opinion among the membership," Leibel explained to her constituents. "We are a small, heterogeneous group whose individual and community needs vary greatly." Careful not to repeat its mistakes from the home birth position statement, the board wanted to assure that a "democratic process was followed" and that members from all regions were consulted.

This was new territory for the ACNM. "No one has yet pressed the Board to 'take a position' on any aspect of the lay midwifery movement," wrote Leibel.[59] "Such a time seems inevitable, and it is now that we urge you to express your concerns—positive, neutral, negative and from a personal and professional point of view."[60] She urged members to write or call her so that she could share their opinions at the next board meeting. Discussion at that 1978 board meeting resulted in the decision to offer an "open forum" on the lay midwifery question at the following ACNM annual meeting. Specific questions were drawn up for members to consider. Should there be an official relationship with lay midwifery groups? Should ACNM be involved with lay midwifery education, certification, or licensure? What would be the risks or benefits of such involvement?[61] No clear agreement could be reached, and the problem would not go away.

Dorothea Lang, president of the ACNM from 1975 to 1977, also sensed that the relationship between nurse and lay midwives would become a divisive issue within the organization. She attended the 1977 El Paso meeting "incognito," afraid that it would jeopardize her standing within the ACNM. "For nurse-midwives, being active in NAPSAC or participating in anything that was outside the ACNM seemed like you were leaving the flock, so to speak," she explained.[62] Like Leibel, Lang's attachment was not to nursing but to midwifery. She fought "tooth and nail" to preserve a faction within ACNM to argue that nurse-midwives were not "extended nurses," nor a "sub-group of nursing." Like many, she questioned whether "nurse" even belonged in the title of the profession. Because she was the president of ACNM, some board members insisted that she never refer to the organization's members as mere "midwives." "I always had to use 'nurse-midwife', or else I would be impeached. So you can tell that the backlash was tremendous, because they knew my philosophy."

Allying with lay midwives proved to be politically divisive. The fact that she attended El Paso incognito underscored this. Lang believed CNMs would fear that she would "walk away with the dynamic core of nurse-midwives" in the divide. "I kept saying, 'There must be another organization.' Since I had been saying that for so long, ACNM was afraid that I might turn the ACNM into something that they didn't want it to be."[63] Lang remained supportive of outreach to non-nurse midwives well after her presidency, as did many CNMs, but determining an organizational platform took years to work out.

At the 1981 ACNM annual meeting, Sister Angela Murdaugh was elected president. That year's open forum continued to focus on whether "nurse" should remain part of a CNMs official title. The organization appeared evenly divided on the issue. But according to Murdaugh, another topic elicited widespread support. "People kept saying, 'We need to be in dialogue with lay midwives. We need to be in dialogue with them.'" When Murdaugh realized there had not been any real substantive dialogue at all, she vowed to get a conversation started.[64]

DIALOGUE DAY

Murdaugh reached out to CNMs who had either started out as lay midwives or had experience working with them, in the hope that they could form a task force for such a dialogue. At the annual NAPSAC conference, she discussed this idea with founder David Stewart, who agreed to help sponsor the dialogue by covering transportation costs. Former La Leche League president Marian Tompson, now executive director of the Alternative Birth Crisis Coalition in Chicago, sent Murdaugh a check for $350 on behalf of her organization.[65]

Murdaugh then consulted with certified nurse-midwives Fran Ventre, Susan Leibel, and Carol Hurzeler on a mid-August conference call. "All agreed that a sit down, face to face conversation was needed between women recognized to be within the lay midwifery movement," she explained. The following week she invited these women to come to Washington, D.C. for an all-day session in October. "I decided to take some aggressive steps toward talking with lay midwives," she explained in a letter to Ina May Gaskin. "Your name was suggested since you are practically a legend in your own time, in midwifery circles. We would like to discuss the importance or non-importance of standards for midwifery education and practice, try to learn more of the strengths that midwifery contains and to see if together we can assume a more assertive role that will assure our survival."[66] Gaskin responded promptly and enthusiastically, noting "it seems that a lot of people worldwide are looking to see what kind of a system we will evolve in this country."[67]

Murdaugh contacted the recently formed Seattle Midwifery School in the hopes that one of its founders could attend the meeting to discuss educational standards for non-nurse midwives. They were too busy, but sent Teddy Charvet as a student representative. Murdaugh also invited lay midwives Helen Jolly, Genna Withrow, and Nancy Mills.[68] All agreed to come. "Words cannot describe the excitement I feel with regard to the prospect of meeting with a group of lay midwives and nurse-midwives for the open dialogue," recalled Helen Jolly, who ran Family Centered Maternity Care in Grand Prairie, Texas. "My mind overflows with thoughts and feelings and ideas about midwifery and the course it's taking in this country."[69]

Word quickly spread about the meeting. One NAPSAC member and nursing student from Boston University read about it in the NAPSAC newsletter. "I am delighted to hear that ACNM is opening an official dialogue with lay midwives of this country," she wrote to Murdaugh. "Lay midwives, who often have a non-medical, non-interventive, home birth outlook, have a great deal to teach our more medical practitioners." Upon further reflection, she thought such a conversation could be "extremely valuable for both sides." Perhaps it could result in some reform of midwifery education in the United States, which she currently found "difficult, time-consuming, and expensive to obtain." Such an alliance "is an important step toward breaking the medical stronghold on the practice of midwifery," she wrote.[70]

On October 30, 1981, four nurse-midwives and four lay midwives sat down at a table together with Murdaugh and a recording secretary to begin the historic conversation. Each midwife introduced herself, describing her background as well as what she hoped could be achieved by the gathering. Murdaugh then stressed the importance of communication while moving forward. What should lay midwives be called, and how could they best be represented? If they were to organize and come up with professional standards, then "lay" would be an inappropriate and potentially misleading term. The group decided to use the term "non-nurse midwife" for the time being, though disagreement over terminology would continue.

The more complex issue was who could assume the term "midwife." What sort of standards needed to be in place? How should they be trained, certified, licensed, and regulated? One participant pointed out that enforcing particular standards would take autonomy away from individual practitioners. "But it was generally accepted," Murdaugh explained, "that it would be the price of credibility."[71] Some non-nurse midwives might prefer to stay underground rather than give up their autonomy. "But the issue is how then can there be credentials and standardization?" Visibility was necessary for survival, as well as credibility.

In many ways, "dialogue day" was really more of a continuation of the key topics of discussion that occurred on the last day in El Paso: What sort of public image to convey (who is a midwife?), how to be represented, how to deal with financial issues, and how midwives should be trained. The difference was in the leadership. In El Paso, the president of the ACNM remained incognito. Four years later in Washington, the president of the ACNM convened the meeting.

Lay midwives needed an organizing body, Murdaugh stressed. And nurse-midwives needed to support them rather than see them as competitors or inferiors. Just as civil rights activist Ella Baker recognized the importance of community empowerment when she encouraged students to form their own civil rights organization (Student Nonviolent Coordinating Committee [SNCC]),[72] Murdaugh sensed that "now is the right time for a new organization."[73] And it would be with ACNM's blessing.

This was an electrifying moment, according to Seattle Midwifery School student representative Therese (Teddy) Charvet, who would become the new organization's first president. Murdaugh announced the need to organize. "And then she just looked at each one of us," remembered Charvet.

"I don't know if everybody had the feeling I did, but I just felt like she zapped me with this mission, to be a part of creating this organization. I was just infused with it . . . I just knew that this was what I should do."[74] It was as if Ann Flower Cumings' message at the opening of the El Paso meeting was coming to fruition. "If you remain true to the battle to get out the truth, the movement will grow, expand and have power."[75]

The group agreed to move forward by planning an open meeting in the spring at the next ACNM conference. Each midwife volunteered to take on part of the work to prepare for the meeting, from writing press releases to hammering out some ideas about education, evaluation, guidelines, and communication. Murdaugh sent a letter to all ACNM members explaining what had transpired on that day, including minutes and a follow up plan.[76]

LEXINGTON AND THE FORMATION OF MANA

Over the next six months, the group of seven prepared for the open meeting, to take place on April 25, 1982, at the ACNM meeting in Lexington, Kentucky. They corresponded about reactions, ideas, concerns, and experiences after the October dialogue. Genna Withrow noted that response to "dialogue day" had been positive in her area, Atlanta. She had received calls "from all over" from "very excited midwives," and she encouraged them to engage in their own "dialogue day" within their own communities.[77]

Carol Hurzeler expressed some concern about backlash from CNMs. A CNM student in Pennsylvania called her to tell her that "all she's heard re our 'group' was anger that ACNM money was used to pay the way for CNM's to go to Washington D.C. to talk to 'them.'" Might all their work actually make the situation worse? "This move might really polarize people! We may get more angry people than helpful ones at our April meeting!"[78] While she was looking forward to Lexington, she wrote that she had a "bit of anxiety re unpleasant confrontations from misunderstandings." [79] Ina May Gaskin responded that she had not run into any negative reactions in Tennessee. "It may exist, but we've heard nothing of it."[80]

All stressed the importance of communication and publicity in order to enhance their visibility. Charvet expressed disappointment "to see so little headline coverage" of the October meeting. She wondered if they "shouldn't rely more on the ole' grapevine to relay the news." Publications took too long to come out, she noted—why not a "chain letter sort of approach, hoping the midwife grapevine would help support the carrying of the news"? If everyone who received a letter made a few copies and sent it on, word would travel "fast and far" and would not cost any individual too much effort or expense.[81] She proposed that Gaskin "start the ball rolling" by using her mailing list from *Mothering*, and the rest of them could follow up with other contacts. "The sooner we get going on it, the more input and interest we will have for our April meeting." Gaskin agreed and also committed to providing headline coverage of the meeting in the next issue of her own midwifery magazine, *The Practicing Midwife*.[82]

Thus, by the time some sixty or seventy midwives gathered on April 25, far more women had joined the conversation than the original group in El Paso. Furthermore, the Lexington organizers recognized the continued importance of dialogue and discussion. After the organizers spoke, the floor was open to anyone in attendance to speak for up to five minutes. The entire meeting was run as a discussion, in order to ensure that anybody who wanted to be heard would be.

Despite all of the organization that went into the meeting, some were disappointed that more had not been done to publicize the event. Marion Donahue noted that "timely communication tools *have* to be used. There were people in this area, in the Kentucky/ Indiana area who did not know about this meeting until last weekend. And it was only after numerous phone calls."[83] Linda Cozzolino, who identified herself as a lay midwife from Kentucky also stressed that they needed to "know about these things ahead of time. I bet there are a lot of midwives who would've loved to be here if they'd had more notice."[84] Fran Ventre, who had agreed back in October to handle communication between CNMs and lay midwives, apologized for "not having carried out her job . . . by making sure the CNM publications were notified of all these happenings."[85] Susan Leibel, who moderated the discussion, noted that "there was a lot of upset among CNMs who are interested in this process who didn't know about the meeting who really want input."[86]

No one wanted to be accused of leaving people out of the decision-making process. Those who had organized events or made policy decisions in the past—such as Daniels and Ventre in planning El Paso, or the ACNM Board in issuing its home birth statement—paid the price for not allowing everyone to weigh in. Backlash had been inevitable.

This time, they tried to be more careful to follow a more democratic procedure, in order to more effectively address the organizational challenges that came up in El Paso. The meeting was tape recorded, so that everyone's comments could be accurately captured. Gaskin took copious notes. Leibel tread cautiously as moderator.

Participants, too, came prepared. Marion Donahue, one of the organizers of the International Childbirth Education Association (ICEA), presented a mission statement that addressed the challenges a new midwifery organization would need to tackle. She believed that visibility was crucial and that the most effective way to increase it was through annual conferences. "You have to have exposure, people have to know who you are, and you have to start promoting yourselves." The group burst into applause as she finished.[87]

Others stressed the need for a national organization to establish licensing guidelines, which would help state groups push for midwifery legislation. A group of Kentucky lay midwives had attempted to get a bill passed through the state legislature. But the state nursing association lobbied "intensely" against them. "Over and over again we were asked for national standards of licensing midwives," one midwife explained. "There must be a national standard; can we follow this? No, there isn't. We could've used support for legislation if there had been regional representatives writing in." The Kentucky midwives had never attempted to write a bill before; feedback from other midwives who had attempted similar legislation would have been helpful, as well as formal approval of the bill from a national organization.[88]

A national organization would also establish credibility. When the Kentucky lay midwives approached the legislature about a midwifery bill, "they didn't even know how to pronounce the word midwifery; they didn't know that we existed, that there was such a thing." A national presence would help to reassure state legislatures that "these weren't a couple of kooks that came up with this idea."[89]

Ruth Beeman, a CNM from Arizona, agreed, stressing the need for national guidelines. She worked as a consultant for the state to organize and supervise home births by licensed midwives. She created the qualifying examinations given to lay midwives in order to get licensure (quite an anomaly), as well as guidelines for clinical practice and continuing education programs. "We have done in Arizona at a state level most of the things you're asking for at the national level." She would have benefited from national standards; instead, she had to use common sense and her own experience to create the state guidelines.[90]

Listeners were stunned, most likely because they were unaware that such guidelines were already in use. They immediately peppered Beeman with questions. How did she come up with guidelines? How did she administer continuing education? Did she have statistics? This was the sort of wisdom and experience that listeners hoped could be applied on a larger scale.

The key, according to Beeman, was to build alliances within the nurse-midwifery and obstetrical communities, rather than to see them as threats. "We have marvelous cooperation between nurse midwives [and] nurse practitioners," she explained. Initially, physicians were concerned, but over the years, many had come around. When the Arizona law was challenged, there was a "coalition of physicians, nurse midwives, nursing, and licensed midwives that really kept the law and made it more responsive to everyone's needs."[91]

Others chimed in with tales of cooperation and support from CNMs. Dorothy Richards introduced herself as a "hillbilly midwife" from rural Kentucky. She explained that when she started delivering babies at home, there were no other midwives from whom she could learn. More recently, she had met some certified nurse-midwives "and I love them," she confessed, laughing. "I think we can work together." Sometimes she found herself relying on their expertise, rather than that of doctors. She hoped that ultimately a new organization would enable them to work together. "I think there's room for both of us."[92] Her comments drew widespread applause, perhaps from the many CNMs in attendance.

But as the conversation continued in a rather unstructured format, the organizers grew increasingly aware of time running out and the enormous tasks left to be done. Cautious not to repeat the mistakes from El Paso, they intentionally privileged an open discussion over a tightly controlled agenda. "Can we get focused, please?" begged Susan Leibel, trying to bring the group together after a break. Someone even suggested turning on a beeper, since that seemed to catch midwives' attention. During the break, Leibel had been approached by midwives wanting to know why organizers hadn't presented a more definitive platform. "Let me be definitive," countered Leibel. "This organization exists. It exists in the mind and the spirit of those who wish it to exist, and it will exist."

How it was to evolve was a different matter, but she could at least offer up a name for the new national organization: The North American Midwives Alliance. Some rumbling came from the audience, at which point Gaskin pointed out the name could always be changed. In fact, it was changed the very next day, when Fran Ventre proposed calling it the Midwives' Alliance of North America, in order to make the acronym MANA, meaning spiritual or divine nourishment.

Leibel's definitive statement helped to push the conversation closer toward the practicalities and priorities of building an organization, including financial considerations. Carol Leonard volunteered to serve as treasurer and do the bookkeeping from her New Hampshire midwifery office. Gaskin volunteered to add extra pages to her quarterly publication, *The Practicing Midwife*, as the official publication of the new organization, at least until it could get on its feet.

In order to build membership, they discussed strategies for promoting MANA and a new public image for lay midwives. Some suggested obtaining mailing lists from consumer organizations, such as NAPSAC, where much of their client base would come from. Ventre suggested developing a flyer to distribute at various meetings related to childbirth, such as childbirth education classes and La Leche League meetings. Charvet suggested the same "chain letter" idea that she had proposed to the original seven organizers.

Then someone asked whether membership would be open to anybody or just midwives. "Everybody," Carol Leonard asserted. "*Levels* of membership," cut in Ventre. But some thought there were already several organizations that welcomed anyone—such as NAPSAC and ICEA. The question was more complicated than it appeared. "Right now we haven't worked out some of the criteria to say who is a midwife," Ventre pointed out. "And that's going to take two or three years to develop." Several people spoke up at once, disagreeing over whether this was the appropriate time to set criteria. Ventre pushed for inclusivity, arguing that it would be problematic to kick people out at a later date because they didn't meet certain standards.

Gaskin agreed, stressing the need to welcome what she called "potential midwives." Most of the mail she received was from people seeking training in midwifery. "I think there are just tens of thousands of women who want training who would be good midwives and that's part of our job is to figure out how we give them a helping hand and introduce them into the profession." And the term itself was undergoing transition. Gaskin was already calling herself a midwife after delivering only four or five babies—"in my head I mean, not publicly, but I knew I was because that was the path I'd chosen." Like many others in the room, she reflected that "it would've been nice to have an organization to relate to at the same time," an organization that would point out educational and networking opportunities. "I think that is part of what this organization can do and I don't think that that will deplete our strength because I think there's such dedication coming from these people that they need to be part of it."[93]

Leibel believed that membership should extend even beyond these "potential midwives" to consumers of midwifery care. She conceived of the organization as not only an "organization *of* midwives" but one that "*supports* midwifery right now." Modern midwifery, born at least in part from the women's health movement, represented a profession on equal footing with its clientele. "This is ultimately where our strength lies, is in the people we serve," Leibel explained. "And I think this organization may be unique in that, as a professional-type organization, it has active participation at some point with the people it serves." Midwifery was a consumer-driven profession. Despite attempts by organized medicine to dismantle it in the United States, midwifery continued to be practiced because of consumer demand.[94] Why not strengthen that alliance—between consumers and their providers—by welcoming them into MANA?

Up until this point of the discussion, participants spoke cautiously about how to move forward, somewhat unsure of the appropriate measures to take or who should take the lead. There had been too many false starts, and no one wanted to be accused of saying the wrong thing. But when Carol Leonard asked if anyone had a "burning need to speak," Linda Irene-Green came forward and changed the tenor of the conversation. "I'm not a midwife and you can all send me away," she prefaced. As an attorney, she represented "more midwives than I'd like to think about."

The room grew intensely quiet, as her firm voice immediately captured full attention. "If you don't stop being so tentative you're going to fold before you start," she warned. It was time to organize and to fight. This was about power, and an alliance of all types of midwives was "absolutely crucial." Keep in mind, she stated frankly, "you're under attack no matter *who* you are."

Irene-Green's tone bespoke her revolutionary message, reminding listeners that their cause was no less important than those of civil rights or other movements fighting discrimination. This was sexism at its worst, and it was time to fight back. "You're under attack by the white male establishment largely because you're women and you're stepping on their toes." That fact had to remain front and center in their consciousness. "You're coming into *their* territory . . . and it's going to make them scream. And it'll be a *little* scream if you step on their toes and a *big* scream if you step on their whole bodies."[95]

Building alliances with other women was therefore essential. All midwives, regardless of title or background, needed to come together to reclaim their rightful place in the birthing chamber. It would not be easy; there would be resistance. "I would just like to see you build yourselves up and see how really important you are and how crucial you are at this stage in the development of health care for women," she stated.

In fact, it was midwives' growing power that was causing the backlash. It had become all too clear to organized medicine that they represented serious competition. "And that's why those doctors are running so hard. Because *they* want to provide that health care for women." And they would do whatever it took to make sure they retained authority. Midwives needed to protect themselves. If anyone in the room was "in any kind of trouble," she urged them to get in touch with her. "You gotta be real careful about denigrating your own status in the legal arena."[96] They were all in this together, after all. "No one kind of midwife is more legal than any other kind of midwife," she argued.

A British midwife in attendance spoke up in agreement, highlighting that this was a uniquely American problem. As an outsider, she found the different terms extremely confusing. "Either you're a midwife, or you're not a midwife," she believed. "You shouldn't be a 'lay midwife' or a 'nurse midwife'. You're a midwife." If there was to be any differentiation at all between midwives, it should be based on location of birth, not the status of the midwife. Was she trained and prepared for the potential emergencies that might happen outside of the hospital? Domiciliary midwives, as they were called in the United Kingdom, needed to be "the most skilled person of all . . . because she's there on her own facing any situation that could appear."[97] Gaskin noted in a letter to her fellow home birth midwives that she "felt like folks appreciated the perspective [the British midwife's] comments gave."[98] Seen in an international perspective, the current (and confused) state of midwifery in the United States appeared outside the norm, raising the possibility that it could be effectively changed.

Critically aware of the time and eager to end with a working plan, moderator Susan Leibel jumped in. "We've gotta take hold of this and be less than ideally democratic and just say we're going to go and do work that has to be done, ok?" She asked the group to support the idea that the "core group" would continue. She welcomed additional volunteers, but knew that there had to be a core group to keep momentum going. "I feel very ambivalent about the whole process, but we've gotta do stuff. It has to be done."[99] The meeting closed with an agreement that they would continue discussions over the course of the week in Lexington, with Ventre offering her hotel room phone number as a place to check in and leave messages.

The following day, the core group met with more CNMs who weren't able to attend the Sunday session. "The room was packed," wrote Gaskin. Former ACNM president Dorothea Lang showed up "very excited." People started writing $25 checks to Carol Leonard. Susan Leibel agreed to serve as interim director, as "everyone seems to feel comfortable with her way of handling meetings." That evening, she dined with the four past presidents of the ACNM to explain the purpose of MANA. Gaskin believed this to be advantageous, noting that Leibel was "pretty diplomatic for how radical she is."[100] In Lexington, they also created a research committee on education and a membership committee, tackling those organizational challenges some had been struggling with since the planning of El Paso.

According to Gaskin, the group had two or three more productive meetings over the course of the week. She found the ACNM conference itself "pretty boring," but expressed satisfaction with the headway she made with some of its established "old guard." "I managed to get straight with Helen Burst, Ruth Lubic and Kitty Ernst, all of whom had been pretty uptight with me," she wrote. "They were glad to know that I appreciated the ACNM's function and that we would be taking special care not to mess up their organization or any of their projects."[101]

At least some ACNM members would understandably have been concerned that a group of lay midwives, some far more radical in their political orientation, had intruded upon their annual conference. "It was interesting to see that Helen [Burst] wasn't bothered by most of my wildest ideas—that midwives should be at the front of the women's peace movement, etc.," reflected Gaskin. "I explained pretty much the same stuff to Kitty and Ruth, and they were very sweet to me (as was Helen at the end of our talk—she hugged me). I told them I thought we needed a radical organization that would cooperate in sisterhood with ACNM."[102] Based on the discussion at the Lexington conference, that appeared to be the case for many midwives who would go on to create and sustain the Midwives Alliance of North America.

"AN INTERESTING AND DIFFICULT POSITION TO OCCUPY"

Yet as Susan Leibel explained to the MANA founders, they were faced with "the challenge of finding compromise points" in the organization's efforts to strengthen midwifery as a profession. She continued to perceive the group as caught between two extremes. "We see ourselves as 'moderates' and as such are viewed by the conservative health care establishment as 'radical' or troublesome," she wrote. At the same time, they were "conversely viewed by the non-traditional/non-licensed health care providers (including many lay-midwives) as leaning dangerously close to the establishment that would coopt/control/destroy midwifery."[It was, as she explained, "an interesting and difficult position to occupy."[103] The messiness of terminology, the infighting, the complications of different and changing laws in different states, and the diversity of background, training, and experience made any organizational position tricky.

These challenges affected not only outsiders' views of MANA, but those within the organization as well. After the meetings in Washington and Lexington, Leibel wrote the other organizers with some reflections. "I saw how we were 'giving birth to' and were accepting responsibility for 'mothering of' an organization." This brought up a range of emotions for her, from excitement and elation to fatigue and fear.[104]

Though Leibel was praised for her excellent job of moderating the Lexington meeting, the fact that she was a CNM worried some members. As much as lay midwife supporters of MANA wanted to see all midwives united, the fact remained that nurse-midwives were insiders in a way that lay midwives would never be. One midwife confided to Gaskin that she had the feeling that Leibel was "not doing much about our new organization and that the leadership should be in the hands of lay midwives if we want to get moving. She has lots of commitments around her own job."[105] Lea Rizack noted "I've always felt the leadership in MANA should be largely lay midwives so that CNMs could not sabotage anything."[106] On the other hand, many felt that having an active CNM presence would help to build alliances and solidify the profession as a whole.

This tension—between trying to create something different from ACNM, and yet also include (or at least ally with) its members—continued to plague the organization. Education and training perpetually divided the groups, making it more difficult to reach compromise. Some certified nurse midwives certainly looked down upon lay midwives, believing them to be unprepared for the job in terms of medical expertise. But many lay midwives looked down upon nurse midwives, suspecting they were unprepared for the job in terms of resisting medical expertise.

This clash over training threatened to undermine MANA's goals. "I do not want to see MANA become an exclusive, elitist organization, admitting to membership only those who are trained in the precise manner which they dictate," wrote Lani Rosenberger in response to MANA president Teddy Charvet's request for a "clearly defined educational process" for lay midwives. Rosenberger interpreted this to mean that apprenticeship training would not "count" as much as a scholastic pathway. "What scares me the most is the parallels to the founding of the AMA in the 1840s," in terms of its impact on those lacking formal credentials.[107] Charvet refuted the charge, suggesting that Rosenberger was "trying to protect yourself and your own sense of validity as a midwife trained by an informal alternative route. You read into my words stuff that just wasn't there."[108] Charvet had recently graduated from the Seattle Midwifery School, where she came to embrace the school's philosophy of standardized education for non-nurse midwives. Yet many within MANA remained opposed to the idea that midwifery training could or should take place in an institutional setting, preferring the more traditional apprenticeship model.

As educational models drew attacks of elitism within MANA, so did financial matters. In the summer of 1983, Gaskin (at that time serving as MANA's VP) received an angry letter from lay midwife Ann Frye regarding an increase in membership fees. In desperate need of funding to stay afloat, the board had decided to raise the fee from $25 to $50 a year, while offering the option of a "non-voting" membership at the original $25.

Frye was aghast, accusing the organization of abusing its power. "It has taken me this many weeks to come to a point where I can at least try to articulate some of the utter outrage I feel about this decision," she wrote. It struck her as "classist, elitist, and extremely male-thinking to assume that those who pay the most money should have the most power." If anything, membership dues needed to be lowered so that it would be more inclusive. The impact, Frye believed, would be to create "a hierarchy of members with the means having most of the power." Those without the funds would most likely drop out of (or never join) the organization because they couldn't afford it. "It would seem my biggest fear is already a reality—'professional midwives'—turning themselves into their own self-serving little cliché; infant-female-ACOG here we come!" She proposed that all members should be given voting privileges and that a sliding scale be introduced, based on income. If MANA continued in this elitist direction, she would withdraw her support. "I DON'T want to become a 'little CNM.'" [109]

Leibel and Charvet were cc'd on the letter, and all three responded defensively to the charges. "I'm sorry you are so fearful of 'professional midwifery' and speak with such anger towards those who are attempting to come to terms with the need to develop their own power bases within the health care system," Leibel wrote. She found Frye's philosophy "equally elitist" in its refusal to acknowledge the current vulnerability of midwives, as well as the need to raise funds. Taking Frye to task for her judgmental tone, she ended her letter by expressing her hope "that the midwives of this continent will stop criticizing each other long enough to share the vision of midwifery care being the 'rule' rather than the 'exception.'"[110] In essence, she was repeating the message articulated by attorney Linda Irene-Green in Lexington. By engaging in infighting rather than alliance building, lay and nurse midwives were losing sight of the real threat of obstetrical power.

Charvet built on this charge in a separate letter to Frye. Did she not understand the precarious position they were in? "We need the support, not the skepticism, of midwives all across the continent if we are going to have the strength to withstand the storm that's brewing up as the medical profession loses its control over the health care system," she wrote. "We midwives need to learn their game and know the political/legal system if we are to protect our profession from going underground again," she warned. Frye's anger was misplaced. "No, we don't want to become an 'infant-female-ACOG' and your name-calling to that effect suggests a bitterness and lack of understanding that should be directed toward ACOG, not your sister midwives."

Like Leibel, Charvet also found Frye's comments elitist. "I don't know what your experience with CNMs has been, but personally I have found many who are sensitive, intuitive midwives, and certainly should not be linked with 'classist, elitist, and extremely male-thinking' philosophies," she wrote. "Unfortunately, it is your own 'elitism' that is creating the problem." Frye needed to "let her prejudices go" and recognize that CNMs were equally invested in protecting midwifery. The ACNM had done "more to restore midwifery into the health care system of this country" than any other organization. While Charvet hoped that MANA might rise to an "even more influential place" than ACNM by giving credibility and training opportunities to all types of midwives, "we have much to thank ACNM for."[111] Attacking the organization would be detrimental to MANA.

Yet Frye was not alone in her concerns that MANA's policies and practices did not go far enough in support of consumer needs or encouraging alternative pathways to licensure (an attack made more frequently against the ACNM). This became a regular source of tension within the organization. It was, perhaps, an inherent problem of building alliances and seeking compromise between medicine and midwifery.

Nowhere was this more apparent than in discussions of race and representation. If MANA was really to represent the more radical arm of midwifery, as Gaskin imagined back at the Lexington meeting, then it needed to focus on building community structures that would empower the disenfranchised, rather than simply provide an alternative for the white middle class. "It is important to acknowledge that the current composition of the midwifery profession in this country is quite unlike the composition of a major segment of the women midwives service, from the perspective of class, race, ethnicity, and native language," wrote a group of Massachusetts midwives and consumers in 1990. One of the justifications for the expansion of midwifery care stemmed from the "deplorable state of maternity care and perinatal outcomes for a large proportion of low-income women, immigrant women and women of color."[112] Yet these were the women least likely to have the means to pay for such care.[113] It was therefore imperative to "address the critical needs of these women by enhancing their participation and self-determination." [114]

In the fall of 1988, the MANA board passed a resolution to provide funding for a seat on the board specifically reserved for a woman of color.[115] "We realized there were midwives who felt MANA was not an organization which could (or cared to) focus on the concerns of their practices and who viewed the organization with a certain amount of skepticism in terms of its ability to accept the different needs of under-represented communities," wrote a member of MANA's Affirmative Action Committee in 1989.[116] "I could see the heart of the people that were involved with MANA, and I saw they had the heart, but they didn't have the experiences with other peoples," observed Sondra Abdullah Zaimah, the first appointed woman of color representative on the board. "What I could see was that midwifery would become a middle class white woman profession, and that it would exclude so many people that needed it as a means of survival." By the late 1980s, MANA had established itself as an organization committed to enhancing the professional status of the North American midwife. "I felt that my original purpose in becoming involved with MANA was to make sure that there was a whole level of folks with another reality involved, and that they wouldn't get forgotten when all these decisions got made," Zaimah explained.[117]

Yet the issue was far from resolved. Midwives of color continued (and still continue) to fight to have their concerns addressed in primarily white professional midwifery organizations. They have insisted that maternity care be addressed within the framework of reproductive justice rather than merely consumer choice. Without access to birth alternatives, women of color, who suffer from disproportionate rates of pregnancy and birth complications, cannot take advantage of the new laws or licensing options that have enabled midwives to make a comeback over the last several decades. MANA's 2012 "I am a Midwife" public education campaign was a step in the right direction, but many believe that MANA and the alternative birth movement more generally have not gone far enough in challenging existing medical, class, and racial hierarchies.

Nonetheless, like many start-up organizations interested in both gaining legitimacy from the mainstream and instituting reforms to current practices, MANA worked to create a balance between the two. Some tasks appeared more challenging than others, particularly in the encouragement of a racially and economically diverse membership and clientele. Yet the women instrumental to MANA's formation faced formidable barriers: lack of money, organizational or legal experience, and access to any real political power. Despite this, they hammered out policies, debated procedures, and fought passionately to defend what they believed was the best way to move midwifery forward.

CHAPTER 6

cᴧɔ

From Professionalization to Education

The Creation of the Seattle Midwifery School

In January of 1979, five women are seated around a table at the Soup and Salad Café in Pike Place Market, Seattle. One orders a pot of tea while the rest pull out textbooks, notes, and a model pelvis, and place them on the table. "Do you think they'll notice this is the third afternoon this week we've had class here?" asks Susan. "It's ok," Marge responds. "I offered the cashier a free pelvic exam. But I think I will ask them to turn the music down a bit when we're ready to start. It was hard to hear last time." The day's "class" is on labor complications, but the instructor, University of Washington obstetrician Durlin Hickok, has not yet arrived. While they wait, the five women hold an impromptu Board of Directors meeting of the Seattle Midwifery School. "Sorry I'm late," announces Hickok, rushing to the table, wearing Groucho glasses as a disguise. "I was afraid I might run into one of my colleagues coming through the market. Now, about shoulder dystocia."

The scene may or may not be an accurate depiction of the actual meeting but it became part of a skit performed annually for incoming students at the Seattle Midwifery School to introduce them to the founders' story. "What was so hysterically funny is that some of us were playing ourselves ten years later or fifteen years later," remembers school founder Suzy Myers. "I've played myself as a young pregnant woman and then with the baby," she chuckles. This scenario quickly captures the unusual circumstances that led to the development of one of the first, and certainly the most influential, schools for non-nurse midwives in the United States. The school's founders– and original Board of Directors—were also the first students. They began with no physical space or money, convincing supportive MDs to tutor them in required subjects. Within fourteen months, and after passing an exam issued by the state Department of Licensing, they were licensed to practice midwifery in the state of Washington. They also ensured that hundreds of women (and a handful of men) could follow in their footsteps.

This chapter traces the development of the Seattle Midwifery School (SMS) from its roots in the feminist Fremont Women's Clinic to a fully accredited direct-entry midwifery program recognized by the U.S. Department of Education. The SMS founders struggled with the same questions of professionalization and cooptation that characterized debates within MANA and the ACNM. Many non-nurse midwives, including some MANA members, adamantly opposed the institutionalization of lay midwifery education. Midwifery was an art as much as it was a trade, they believed, and imposing standards such as a core curriculum might threaten their distinctiveness (as well as exclude those who were less educationally and economically privileged). How to create a system of midwifery training that would legitimize and protect their trade without stepping on any toes proved to be enormously challenging.

The history of the SMS is as surprising as it is remarkable, however, because the women who founded the school did not set out to do so. Like many lay midwives of the mid-1970s, they were adamantly opposed to the structure and function of organized medicine and its monopoly on women's bodies. They therefore had no interest in replicating any part of its system, including medical education and licensure. They joined the chorus of critical consumers and alternative practitioners who voiced a "crisis of confidence" in modern medicine. As social critic Ivan Illich argued in 1976, the medical establishment had become a "major threat to health." Providing doctors with the exclusive right to define, regulate, and practice modern medicine, the "university-trained bourgeoisie" needed to be restrained by a grassroots lay movement that would reclaim control over "medical perception, classification, and decision-making."[1] Medical power needed to be restored to the people.[2]

When the SMS founders first became lay midwives in the mid-1970s, they utilized the rhetoric of social critics such as Illich. They expressed disdain for the socially destructive power of medical licensure. "It seems to us that [licensure] protects not primarily the public, but the medical profession itself, at the expense of the public," they declared.[3] Deliberately positioning themselves as outsiders, they opposed the system of licensing "that controls who's trained, what they learn, and how they are able to use that knowledge" and wanted no part of it for the training or practice of midwifery.[4]

But between 1975, when they formed a birth collective, and 1978, when they incorporated the Seattle Midwifery School, the founders' position radically shifted. Three hundred home deliveries and a changing social climate facilitated that shift. As the women gained experience and confidence that they were serving a need in the community, they sought the protection and legitimacy that licensure could provide. Their experiences over the course of the decade reveal the developing political consciousness of these self-proclaimed feminists interested in changing birth practices.

SEATTLE'S ALTERNATIVE HEALTH MOVEMENT

When SMS founder Suzy Myers arrived in Seattle in 1971, newly graduated from Clark University, she quickly discovered that the city was a "hotbed for the free clinic movement."[5] There were seventeen alternative free clinics in Seattle in 1971, serving approximately fifty thousand patients per year.[6] By 1971, over 150 such clinics—typically storefront operations offering basic medical services in poor neighborhoods—had opened up in largely urban areas nationwide.[7] In Seattle, they included the Fremont Women's Clinic, Country Doctor, and the Open Door clinic. "I hooked up with a group of people who were trying to start a new one called the Fremont Women's Clinic so I got in on the ground floor," she recalled. The clinic was developed by residents of the Fremont-Ballard-Wallingford-Queen Anne neighborhoods in 1971. It was one of only two clinics that offered gynecological services for women, in addition to general preventive health care services for neighborhood male and female residents.[8]

Jo Anne Myers-Ciecko arrived in the Seattle area in 1974 with her husband. Through some of his college friends, she got involved in a group called the People's Health.[9] "I had been part of this collective, political collective, and had been doing health care kind of organizing support work around the community clinics here in Seattle," she recalled in a 1999 interview.[10] "It started up as a support network for the free clinics around town and started getting into organizing health care workers and defending the public health hospital, which was under siege at that point." She discovered a passion for women's health that would lead her to the Fremont Women's Clinic as a client.

When SMS founder Marge Mansfield arrived in Seattle in 1972, she immediately noticed the impact of the free clinic movement on the city's social landscape. She had lived in Seattle with her family when she was in high school, then left the area to attend college in Colorado and spend a year in Europe before returning. The sheer number of community clinics that had emerged during her absence left her awestruck. "It was so strong, and we knew that that was part of a national movement, that there were community clinics in other cities, and the whole, you know, demystifying medicine and taking it back to the people, you know, pelvic parties, and all that stuff."[11] Mansfield's observation attests to the increasing prominence of health as a topic that affected everyone, regardless of age, gender, race, or income.

Mansfield's introduction to the community clinic movement was as a patient at the Aradia Women's Health Center. The center opened its doors in April of 1972 to provide gynecological care for all women "regardless of socioeconomic status, race, ethnicity, or sexual orientation." However, the center largely served the residents of its predominantly white neighborhood located near the University of Washington.[12] The founders did attempt to address issues of race and racism, participating in a workshop hosted by the Third World Women's Resource Center in 1973 designed to "increase their sensitivity and responsiveness to the reproductive health needs of women of color."[13] The clinic provided contraception (pills, IUDs, and diaphragms), pap smears, venereal disease screening, and health education, encouraging patients to be actively involved in their own health care.[14] In an effort to eradicate existing medical hierarchies (as well as to provide affordable care), most services were provided by "paras," feminist community health workers, or paramedics without medical degrees.[15]

When Mansfield visited and learned she had an abnormal pap smear, she was struck by the difference in treatment compared to the first pelvic exam she had experienced in the Netherlands with an ob/gyn. "The way they handled my abnormal pap smear and getting the cervix frozen and all that, and the TLC and the calls back and all that, I mean, it was just good stuff." In the end, Aradia didn't just reassure her about her own health; it inspired her to completely rethink the politics of health care.

Until her Aradia visit, Mansfield had wanted to become a doctor. But her experience with feminist paramedics at Aradia made her realize a desire to practice a more alternative style of medical care, one that was explicitly feminist. She had a friend who worked at the Country Doctor clinic and learned that they were doing paramedic training. "I learned about the community clinic thing, and that really struck a chord. I just really felt that was something I should look into." Country Doctor was one of the first community clinics located downtown, in the Capitol Hill neighborhood, where 75 percent of the residents did not have access to health care. Because Mansfield was not a Capitol Hill resident, she was not allowed to train there. Instead, the staff suggested she investigate the Fremont Clinic closer to her home, where she began working in 1973. There she would meet Suzy Myers and later Jo Anne Myers-Ciecko (whose baby she would deliver at home). "It wasn't specifically midwifery that drew me," she explained. "It was the whole thing very personal, and just, you know, the demystifying the whole process, you know. All those ideas that characterized the popular health movement in those days."[16]

The growing popularity of home birth in the Seattle area generated interest, as well as some concern, among locals. In 1971, the *Seattle Post-Intelligencer* published a special four-part series on "Babies Born at Home." The new phenomenon of young couples opting to stay out of the hospital was not limited to Chicago, Washington D.C., or Santa Cruz. "Can this be Seattle, 1971?" asked journalist Judi Moore. "It is, and the woman is not alone in her choice to give birth in her own bed rather than a clinic or hospital." The numbers were small (50 home births in Seattle-Kings County in 1969), but growing, indicative of a burgeoning consumer movement.[17]

Just who was attending these births appeared to be in question in the early 1970s. Although the state of Washington had a midwifery law on the books from 1917, no one had attempted to apply for licensure in decades. Health professionals gathered at a conference sponsored by the University of Washington School of Nursing to discuss the issue in 1972. The title of the conference, "Meeting the Consumer Challenge—Home Birth in the 70's," suggested the extent to which this was a consumer-driven trend requiring greater attention on the part of birth practitioners. According to Jo Anne Myers-Ciecko, panelists and topics did not address the presence of home birth lay midwives, instead focusing on the handful of male physicians involved.[18] Newspaper coverage of home birth in Seattle in the early 1970s also highlighted male physicians' role. As in other parts of the country, lay midwives remained largely under the radar, often working under the direction of the few physicians who were willing to risk their reputation by training them.

By 1976, state vital statistics suggested that home birth was more than just a passing trend and that meeting the consumer challenge was more urgent than ever before. The number of non-hospital births more than quadrupled between 1968 and 1976 (213, rising to 1,045). "Home Deliveries Aren't Just a Fad," noted the *Seattle Post-Intelligencer* in 1976. Dr. Stanley Harris "never intended to go into home deliveries but was talked into it by patients who were determined to have their babies at home," noted reporter Judi Hunt. After agreeing to home deliveries four years earlier, by 1976, half of his clients gave birth at home. "It isn't going to go away," noted Dr. Morris Gold, who had been doing home deliveries for 28 years. "So, rather than pretend that it might, we ought to be finding ways to make it easier for these insistent young parents to have their children at home with medical assistance. Otherwise, they will do it anyway. And without the experienced hands of physicians or trained health-care providers."[19]

Dr. Gold's warning came perhaps too late. The number of out-of-hospital births being attended by someone other than a doctor or nurse increased by nine times, to 523 births in 1976.[20] Fewer local doctors were available or willing to deliver at home. That year, Dr. Jim Campbell, in charge of the home birth services at the Country Doctor clinic, moved away. Suzy Myers remembers Campbell as a "total hippie . . . he was just you know he was really out there." He was "purposefully provocative," talking to medical residents about the simplicity of birth, wearing torn up jeans and a t-shirt.[21] Five women, including Jackie Mertz, worked with him over a two-year period, attending over 100 births.[22] The home birth group "kind of collapsed without him."[23]

While Mertz was delivering babies at home for Country Doctor, Marge Mansfield and Suzy Myers were doing well-woman gynecological care at Fremont. "I loved it," remembered Mansfield. Her instincts after visiting Aradia had proven correct. "I liked learning more stuff all the time, just learning more gynecology. It was really interesting."[24] Myers remembered feeling like there was "a little dose of magic, I'm going to just say, something that is really not explicable, [that] happened around birth and midwifery." As a women's health activist, she felt something "potent and powerful about putting a speculum in a woman's vagina." She was not yet involved in childbirth, but her friend Jackie Mertz was. Mertz would tell her what she was seeing and learning at Country Doctor: "And I was like, I was just completely drawn to it. I could not get enough of the birth stories. . . . That was it, that was what I wanted to do. I don't even know why. I can't explain it to you. I had never seen a birth."[25]

THE FREMONT BIRTH COLLECTIVE

Then, the opportunity presented itself. When Dr. Campbell left Country Doctor, Jackie Mertz moved over to the Fremont Clinic, and ideas started percolating about how to continue a home birth practice through Fremont. As the Fremont group explained later, Country Doctor's home birth practice "laid a lot of the ground-work for us."[26]

On February 14, 1975, a group of individuals interested in developing a home birth service under the auspices of the Fremont Women's Clinic held a meeting in the clinic's examining room. Anyone was invited to attend, and eighteen people showed up, including two young long-haired, alternative-minded doctors, Tom Artzner and Steve Gloyd. Gloyd was doing a residency in family medicine at the time, and Artzner had completed an internship. Neither of them had witnessed a home birth, but had some experience with hospital birth.[27] "I just went, YES!" Myers remembers. "Let's do it!"[28] The group decided to form a birth collective, which would include Myers, Mansfield, Mertz, the two doctors, and two others who worked at

Fremont, Susan Rivard and Miriamma Carson. In the skit version of this meeting, props included an Indian bedspread backdrop, patchouli incense, and a copy of Ina May Gaskin's *Spiritual Midwifery*, which had just been published. The founders wanted to make students aware of their countercultural origins.

First on the agenda was to educate themselves. The group studied obstetric textbooks from the University of Washington Health Sciences Library. Mertz became the primary teacher of home births, but the doctors trained the women as well. Suzy Myers recalls how "unbelievably grateful" she was to Gloyd "for being brave enough to do what he did on our behalf . . . he was an amazing teacher."[29] By June, the group felt they had successfully acquired some basic theoretical knowledge of obstetrics and prenatal care.

In September, they began attending home births. After each one, members reviewed all the details of labor and delivery "so it was a learning experience" for all of them. Within a year, members had participated in the delivery of 120 babies. One of the two doctors supervised the first seventy or eighty, "gradually moving more into the background until the midwives had become adequately trained to meet most complications."[30] The midwives kept careful records of all births, presenting their findings at a NAPSAC conference in 1977. Their clientele, they explained at the meeting, came from a wide variety of economic and political backgrounds—from "counterculture folks and working class people," to professionals, including obstetrical nurses and childbirth educators.[31]

The Fremont Birth Collective adopted the philosophy of the larger Fremont Women's Clinic, as well as that of all feminist women's health clinics of the 1970s.[32] As part of a desire to challenge the power and authority of organized medicine, these clinics were anti-hierarchical and run by lay women rather than health professionals. If it worked effectively in a women's health clinic, as Mansfield felt it had at the Aradia Women's Health Center, why not at a birth clinic? "All aspects of clinic work are done by lay paramedics who have been trained primarily at the clinic and have studied on their own," members of the Birth Collective wrote. "We have not attended professional schools; we are not certified or licensed." This was intentional; they had established the clinic "to present a model of non-alienating, non-hierarchical relationships both between 'patient' and health care worker and among health workers themselves."[33] To feminist health activists, it was crucial to collapse the boundaries between health care provider and patient in order to demystify medicine and empower women to "take their bodies back."[34] They saw it as a revolutionary process and one that required that they maintain their status as lay, rather than professional, midwives. "Until such a political system is built in which people have real power and control over their health care, we see no reason to buy a piece of

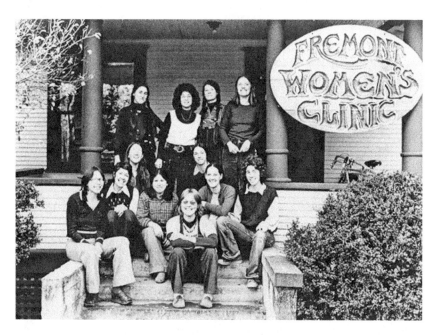

Figure 6.1 Fremont Women's Clinic, ND. Suzy Myers personal collection.

the medical profession for ourselves."[35] It was important to maintain their status as outsiders.

Many of these Fremont birth activists had cut their teeth in New Left and civil rights organizations while in college, crediting these formative experiences as influencing their later involvement in women's health.[36] "All through high school I had been an activist in the civil rights movement," Suzy Myers recalls. She had been a member of SNCC and protested the Vietnam War. "I was marching in the streets, we shut down the university, I mean, I was an activist. I got arrested." Her activist tendencies continued after she moved to Seattle. What sparked her interest in the Fremont collective "was not from the point of view of being a practitioner. That wasn't what interested me. It was more about how to change the world, through health care reform."[37] Civil rights and New Left organizations promoted the idea that revolutionizing health care could transform race and class-based hierarchies and empower minorities and the poor. Their actions inspired many college-aged women of the sixties to hope the same strategy could work to liberate women.[38]

Jo Anne Myers-Ciecko was also inspired by social movements of the 1960s. "We were also all very much engaged in various aspects of the movements for social change," she recalled. As a young person, she remembered being very engaged in civil rights and ideas about inequities and injustice, along with "the idea that you could change things. I mean, that's a very powerful thing, you could change things." While attending Oregon State University, she found it was "attractive to be engaged in the opposition to the [Vietnam] war."[39] She did "all kinds of radical organizing stuff at Oregon State" protesting the war.[40] "Those were powerful, potent experiences at a time of life when a lot of formative stuff happens anyway," she pointed out. "And then the women's movement for me kind of came in around the anti-war stuff." She helped to start a women's liberation speakers bureau in college. "Somehow or other we had gotten it together that there was this other facet to our work which was not just anti-war work and not just environmental activist work, because we were starting to get into that, too, but then also this other side of it, which was the women's stuff."[41] In the end, it was the "women's stuff"—specifically, childbirth—that would become her passion and her profession.

Coming of age in the late 1960s and being engaged with social justice issues while in college contributed to these women's approach to midwifery and medicine. "We had a vision for a better world that was predicated on a revolution," Suzy Myers explained.[42] And that enabled them to make demands of the medical system that previously would have been unimaginable. "We were pretty brazen about it, you know," remarked Mansfield. "I don't know if I would have had [the chutzpah] if I wasn't in the clinic."[43]

They also became more intrepid as they gained experience. Their very first client was one of their own: Suzy Myers, who was already pregnant when they formed the Birth Collective in 1975. "And therefore the guinea pig everybody was practicing on," she recalls. The birth did not, however, go as expected. She had a forty-hour labor, eventually transferring to the hospital. "I was so completely naïve I never even thought about going to the hospital," she said. She had no health insurance. "I never even considered that I might need to go to the hospital." But after two days of agony she felt ready to get it over with. She was admitted to University Hospital with her partner, along with Steve Gloyd, MD, Jackie Mertz as her midwife, and Marge Mansfield as her assistant.

Out of their element, the power dynamics immediately shifted. "You know, everything changed when we got to the hospital," Mansfield remembered. "It was really foreign and yucky." Suzy pushed for two hours, at which point the resident obstetrician wheeled her into the delivery room. Besides her partner, only Gloyd was allowed in; the rest were made to wait outside, including Suzy's appointed midwife.

Perhaps it was best that they were not permitted to enter, for what they would have witnessed certainly would have horrified them. As Myers' labor progressed, the doctors prepared to enlarge the vaginal opening with a surgical cut. Episiotomies had become standard procedure in the delivery room by the mid-twentieth century; by 1980 they were performed in 60 percent of all deliveries (far higher for first-time mothers), ostensibly to prevent tearing.[44] But later studies questioned the utility and safety of the procedure, particularly the mediolateral (rather than the midline) cut. One study concluded that "the incision substantially increases maternal blood loss, the average depth of posterior perineal injury, the risk of anal sphincter damage and its attendant long-term morbidity, the risk of improper wound healing, and the amount of pain in the first several postpartum days."[45] Most midwives involved in home births did not believe such a procedure was needed, advocating other methods to stretch the perineum.

Thus when Gloyd heard the resident instruct the attending physician to "cut a big medio-lateral episiotomy so that you have enough room," his jaw dropped. "Steve knew what that meant," Suzy explained. "I was crippled for six months." The resident then used an early prototype of the vacuum extractor to suction the baby out. Suzy described it as "horrible"; the vacuum cup looked "like a toilet plunger. . . I mean they must have thought I was going to deliver some kind of a moose." She describes the experience as "really awful." [46] Like Jo Anne Santana, Raven Lang, and so many others before her, Myers discovered that her traumatic hospital delivery furthered her conviction that childbirth was in dire need of reform.

Myers' birth experience galvanized the group to demand changes in hospital policy. "I didn't understand anything about hospital birth at the time," Mansfield later explained, and others probably agreed.[47] Focused on creating the right support and setting for a home birth, they had neglected to think through what might happen when they needed to transfer care to the hospital.

FROM SUCCESSFUL TO STRAINED: RELATIONS WITH HOSPITAL STAFF

The Fremont Birth Collective midwives realized that in addition to providing their clients with competent and comfortable care at home, they needed to plan for smooth, coordinated care if hospital transfer was needed. They noted that Country Doctor's birth service had had a "less-than-optimal relationship" with Seattle hospitals and that many lay midwives "are so underground as to have *no* relationship." Members of the Fremont group had also had some bad experiences, and so "have approached several area hospitals to inform them assertively of what we're doing."[48] They didn't ask; they simply informed. Galvanized by successes within the consumer/patient's rights movements (such as the establishment of the Patient's Bill of Rights in 1973, by the AHA), the Fremont group felt increasingly entitled to make demands of the medical profession. They saw themselves, as did many consumer-driven health groups of the 1970s, as watchdogs, there to protect the best interest of the patient.[49]

Sometimes, it worked. While neither Mertz nor Mansfield were allowed to be in the room during Myers' delivery, they ultimately convinced University Hospital to modify its policy. In December of 1975 the administrative nursing supervisor announced updated hospital guidelines on their behalf. "Obstetrical patients from the Fremont Clinic who have planned to have a home delivery, and are referred to University Hospital for delivery, may be accompanied during labor and delivery by: 1. A labor companion (i.e., baby's father or a friend) and 2. One health-care-giver from the Fremont Clinic (i.e., physician, lay-midwife, or medical assistant.)"[50] This was an impressive coup; rarely were lay midwives permitted to accompany a client into the delivery room.[51]

Some University Hospital doctors responded remarkably courteously to the midwives' demands. Dr. Zane Brown, the director of perinatal medicine, thanked the Birth Collective for the feedback of their patients who had delivered at University Hospital in 1977. "This has been most helpful in adjusting obstetrical practice in this Hospital to the changing needs and attitudes of the public." Part of this adjustment had resulted in reconfiguring the hospital delivery rooms to "hopefully more nearly approximate the home environment." In new "short-stay" rooms, women would be admitted, labor, deliver, and recover in the same room. "The décor will be 'homey' and the charges hopefully will be commensurate with the limited hospital services provided."[52] One can imagine that this was hardly the compromise that the Fremont Birth Collective was looking for.[53] But Brown's acknowledgment of the "changing needs and attitudes of the public" indicated his awareness that 1970s consumers were far more vocal in their demands than previous generations had been. Now, they had somewhere else to go.

In a surprising move, Brown not only tolerated the midwives' presence, he welcomed it. "You are certainly welcome to attend all OB departmental conferences whether your patients are the topic of discussion or not," he wrote. He could not guarantee a "uniform reception to the midwife attending a patient transferred to the hospital," due to the high volume of obstetrical residents. Yet he believed most of his residents were "concerned and polite" and would respond "most appropriately" if introduced.[54] This unusual gesture undoubtedly improved relations between lay midwives, their clientele, and University Hospital staff. Perhaps Brown's conciliatory tone was strategic, as he sensed that power dynamics, though still in the hospital's favor, were beginning to shift.

Hospital patients played an important role in shaking up hospital hierarchy. As consumers were encouraged to "shop" for the right doctor or midwife, their expectations of gentle and respectful treatment increased. They were therefore more willing to complain when their expectations were not met. One woman, for example, was admitted to the emergency room at University Hospital because of an unproductive labor at home. She was given an IV and hooked up to a fetal monitor for observation. Two male doctors performed several exams on her over the next few hours. She described one as "extremely rude, impersonal and unprofessional." He apparently did not warn her that he was going to do an internal exam. "He then proceeded to roll my bed down flat, with no warning, as quickly as possible, and in the middle of one of my contractions. His next move, while I was still in contraction and in pain from having my bed so quickly rolled down, was to pull my legs apart for me, since I wasn't moving fast enough, and to perform the roughest, most painful vaginal exam I've ever had." Later, she learned that the doctor apologized to her husband for his behavior, rather than directly to her, which only served to heighten her anger and disappointment in how she was treated. "I cannot stress too much the negative effect of Dr. X's exam on my confidence in the staff at University Hospital."[55]

But it was diplomacy, rather than fury, that prompted her to write. Perhaps a meeting with the hospital administrator was in order. "I am anxious that University Hospital continue its flexibility in alternative birth methods and if my observations can help in any way please contact me."[56] If home birth was an increasingly popular trend, and University Hospital was known for its flexibility with emergency transfers, why risk that reputation with rudeness? Midwives and their clients would simply turn to a different hospital for support.

As they became more outspoken in their demands, however, they triggered a backlash. In February of 1978, the Birth Collective demanded a meeting with the director of diagnostic ultrasound in the Department of Radiology after several of their home birth clients complained about poor treatment. Written in a somewhat condescending tone, the midwives pointed out the importance of open communication and mutual feedback between midwives, clients, and hospital staff. They felt "very positively" about their meetings with the nursing staff and Dr. Brown in the hospital's obstetrical department.

The same could not be said for the staff of the diagnostic ultrasound clinic, where their request for a meeting with a doctor was denied. "We consider her refusal to hear criticism as a direct statement of her unwillingness to respond to the people she's 'serving,'" they wrote. "As a health care provider this arrogance is intolerable." Confident of their power to influence the consumer marketplace, they ended their letter with a threat. Unless they could be assured that clientele referred for ultrasound would not have to see that particular doctor, the Collective midwives would send them elsewhere.[57]

The director of diagnostic ultrasound provided no attempt to placate the midwives or take their demands seriously. He explained that the "very full daily schedule" of patients requires that they arrive on time for their appointments with a full bladder "in order to obtain a diagnostic exam." If patients do not sit still during the exam, "the images produced will be blurred and therefore a waste of everyone's time and effort." Ensuring all patients receive "the best care" required their full cooperation.[58] The real problem was not disrespectful doctors, he suggested; it was noncompliant patients. Of course, this mindset was exactly what had prompted these women to opt out of hospital birth in the first place. The situation was worse at other area hospitals. In late 1976, for example, one of the Collective's pregnant clients had to do an emergency transfer to St. Peter Hospital in Olympia, about an hour southwest of Seattle. Unhappy with her experience there, she filed a grievance against the attending obstetrician and the hospital. Not only was her grievance denied, but both she and Dr. Artzner also received excoriating letters from the Chair of the Grievance and Ethics Committee, Dr. Angela Bowen. "The committee was unanimous in feeling that the hospital had discharged it's [sic] responsibility adequately," she wrote to the client. Disturbed by the nature of the case, she brought it to the local medical society for further discussion, summarizing the society's response. "There is genuine concern that home delivery in the absence of experienced and well trained people puts both mother and child at inexcusable risk," she wrote to the client. "We therefore urge you to reconsider your alternatives and direct your energy toward providing a health care facility that more nearly meets your ideals and still provides every practical safety for mother and child. A tragedy in this area will be of monumental proportions to all involved when it occurs."[59] Why the client should be responsible for the provision of a health care facility is not clear. The Chair wrote a separate letter to Artzner (who by implication she found neither experienced nor well trained), chiding him as well. "If you wished to continue the care yourself you could have requested a temporary staff privilege," she wrote. She also took the opportunity to share remarks of several physicians who disapproved of Artzner's use of Pitocin in home births, considering it unsafe in view of the potential for "potential life-threatening adverse reactions."[60]

Bowen's jab at Artzner underscored the hostility that many home birth doctors experienced from hospital-based obstetricians, even in cities that appeared to welcome alternative lifestyles and practices such as Seattle and Santa Cruz. By 1977, backlash against the Fremont Birth Collective's doctors had escalated. "Until recently the harassment we'd been feeling had been only in the form of innuendos and slanderous comments," clinic members wrote. "But recently we've been experiencing harassment in the form of an attack on the licensed doctors." Years later, Myers reflected on how much worse it could have been: "I'm amazed [Gloyd] didn't get thrown out of his residency," she said, noting how brave he was and what a risk he took.

The midwives, too, were taking risks. Unlicensed, perhaps they had less to lose than Gloyd or Artzner. But as they gained notoriety and visibility, they were increasingly likely to get into legal trouble. They knew that Washington state law "forbids 'aiding and abetting' those practicing medicine or midwifery without a license."[61] In June of 1977, they sent out a letter informing all clients and potential clients of their legal vulnerability. "An important thing to consider is that in spite of what we feel is a very responsible attitude toward our training and representing the extent of our skills to people coming to us, we are illegal. It is against state law to practice midwifery without a license, or assist those who do," they wrote.[62]

Someone apparently forwarded a copy of the letter to state officials. In July of 1977, the collective received a letter from Roz Woodhouse, director of the Department of Licensing, summoning them to Olympia to discuss their unlicensed midwifery practice. "We thought, she's going to throw us in the slammer, you know?" remembers Suzy Myers. "I mean I literally said goodbye to my family, being a drama queen. I said I don't know when we're going to come back from this meeting. They may just put us in handcuffs, you know?"[63] According to Mansfield, they drove down to Olympia with Steve Gloyd and a lawyer friend to meet with Woodhouse and a representative from the Attorney General's Office. She remembers feeling vulnerable. "I mean, we were, yeah, in a sketchy position. Not a whole lot to say about that."[64] Myers and Mansfield were well aware of the 1973 bust in Santa Cruz, as well as the legal trouble many other unlicensed midwives had gotten into in the years since. Why should their situation be any different?

Much to their surprise, Woodhouse treated them with "warmth and grace."[65] She was "so friendly and really nice," Mansfield recalled.[66] Woodhouse had just that year been appointed director of the Department of Licensing by the governor, becoming the first female Chief Motor Vehicle Administrator in the nation, as well as the first African-American woman to hold a cabinet level position in Washington State.[67] She would later become the first female CEO of the Seattle Urban League.[68]

She also happened to have a sister who was a nurse-midwife. "We walk into her office and she says 'how can I help you? Let's figure this out.' And we were dumbstruck, our mouths were hanging open." The problem was that the 1917 midwifery law stipulated that in order to become licensed to practice, a person must have graduated from an "incorporated school of midwifery in good standing" and pass an exam given by the state. As the Birth Collective midwives pointed out, there were no schools of midwifery in the state (or any other) for non-nurse midwives.

In August, the midwives sent Woodhouse a three-page single-spaced letter describing the extensive training and practice they had received through the Fremont Birth Collective. They described didactic courses, prenatal clinics, and on-the-ground training at home births. For example, "both the trainee and the doctor performed the internal exams," and "progress of labor was discussed by all involved." Washington state law stipulated that midwifery training must take place over two calendar years with at least seven months of study in each year, but they had already done that. "We feel this constitutes a thorough, albeit ongoing training program," they argued. Their training "should be recognized as valid," thereby permitting them to take a licensing exam given by the state. "To not allow people like us access to a reasonable test where we might demonstrate our competency gained through supervised instruction and practice clearly perpetuates and reinforces the monopoly and control in the medical profession."[69] Woodhouse would not allow them to take the exam, instead proposing that the midwives start an incorporated school to "train midwives registered under the Proprietary School Act."[70] In the meantime, they needed to stop practicing midwifery illegally.

Woodhouse's decision elicited a mixed reaction from the Fremont midwives. Mansfield noted that suspending their practice was disheartening, but probably inevitable, given the vulnerable position they were in. On the other hand, they were excited about the idea of starting a school. "We felt righteous about it and felt like we could put together the best school in the world," she reflected.[71] Myers believed the decision was a defining moment in their history. "If not for her, who knows?" she asked. "Who knows what our story would have been? Probably a minor, a very minor homebirth collective of hippy women at a Fremont women's clinic who did home births. So what?"[72]

FOUNDING THE SEATTLE MIDWIFERY SCHOOL

Over the next few months, members of the Birth Collective brainstormed over how to build a school, noting it was going to be "a long and difficult project to launch." They needed to think about the nuts and bolts—curriculum, staffing, and fundraising—along with philosophy and vision. Given their politics, how could they ensure that their pathway to licensure did not replicate the very system they were fighting against? "We had studied and discussed the issue of professional licensing quite a bit, considering it historically to be a mechanism of cooptation by the medical establishment," they explained.[73] "We envision a school that not only offers fine technical training, but does it with the right orientation of non-interference in birth and respect for the process. We want the school to promote non-hierarchy and avoid the many negative traits of professional medicine."[74] Deciding they were up for the task, they incorporated the Seattle Midwifery School in May of 1978.

Mansfield focused on developing curriculum and trying to "drum up teachers." Among them were Durlin Hickok, the obstetrician portrayed in the SMS skit at Pike Place Market, and Katherine Camacho Carr, a certified nurse-midwife who had just opened a birth center in Seattle. Both volunteered to teach them free of charge. Susan Anemone worked on grant writing, and the others did "a little bit of everything."[75]

Their intention was to create a program similar to existing nurse-midwifery programs, minus the nursing requirement. In order to do so, they had to convince Department of Licensing director Roz Woodhouse that the school would fill an existing need. With that in mind, they solicited letters of support from certified nurse-midwives who had reviewed their curriculum proposal. CNM Katherine Camacho Carr noted the "great interest in the Seattle area and throughout the Northwest for the development of a school of midwifery," as well as a "need for non-physician birth attendants . . . consumers are calling for their services."[76] Another CNM, Elaine Schurmann, believed the proposed curriculum to be a "comprehensive program of study" and noted her willingness to accept Seattle Midwifery students and serve as preceptor, as well as provide lectures on nursing and midwifery.[77] "The need of more qualified practitioners is evident."[78] Rosemary Mann, director of the Nurse-Midwifery Education program at the University of California, San Francisco, noted that the concept of midwifery training without the prerequisite of professional nursing was of "great interest" to her. "I am convinced that the effort to identify those nursing skills inherent in midwifery with the goal of encompassing those skills in a Midwifery Curriculum is worth investigating," she wrote. She expressed her support and satisfaction with the curriculum developed by the SMS.[79] Given the sometimes antagonistic relations between lay and nurse midwives, and conflicts over professional organization, it is significant that the SMS was able to gain the support of these notable CNMs.

A handful of local doctors also provided support for the proposed curriculum. George Hibbs believed it to be comparable to nurse-midwifery programs and expressed willingness to serve on the faculty as well as their advisory board. "Midwifery is here, and needs the academic and legal status to make it a recognized and valuable part of the health care delivery system," he wrote. "I support it as an idea whose time has come."[80] Obstetrician Philip DuBois "heartily endorse[d] the concept and [saw] the well-trained, licensed midwives as valuable obstetrical care providers. Since there are no midwifery schools in the Seattle area at present, I urge the facilitation of a quality program."[81] Interestingly, in the copy he sent to the midwives, he penciled an apology on the back for the delay, explaining he was "unsure at first as to where I stood with this." [82] Perhaps he wasn't endorsing it as "heartily" as suggested in the letter.

Two doctors from University Hospital, where the midwives regularly took clients needing to transfer to the hospital, also expressed ambivalence. Dr. Marcia Coleman felt unable to condemn or endorse the establishment of the school. "However, I will state that these women have filled a need for alternative care," she acknowledged. "Such care will continue to be sought by a certain segment of our population, no matter what care is provided by established medical facilities. It is important that we attempt to provide that group with well-trained practitioners."[83] Dr. Zane Brown, who on previous occasions told the midwives they could call on him any time, "day or night," for help, was in this instance not able to provide it.[84] He sought approval from the chair of the Department of Obstetrics and Gynecology at the University of Washington, who felt that his department and the university "could not support the program or its curriculum at this time." The chair believed that any communication with the state Department of Licensing would be "inappropriate."[85]

Steve Gloyd did not find such a response surprising. "I imagine you have already encountered (or will) some resistance to the school from organized medicine and nursing, whose turf such a school would invade," he wrote to Woodhouse. He described the medical profession as "tight and elitist" with "strong vested interests and barriers to entry that are difficult for ordinary working people to surmount." Midwives, after all, could potentially put obstetricians out of business.

But even were it not for economic considerations, many medical professionals were uncomfortable with the idea of training "otherwise non-medical people" to become independently practicing midwives. He, too, initially had reservations as to whether it would be safe or beneficial. But his three years of training lay midwives convinced him that it was indeed "quite possible" to "very adequately" train someone without any previous experience to become a midwife within one to two years. The training at the Fremont Birth Collective, though "considerably less sophisticated and organized" than the proposed SMS program, had been highly effective.[86]

Perhaps more importantly, it filled two urgent needs: unlicensed midwives needed more training, and home birth consumers needed more protection. Gloyd estimated that there were probably over one hundred people practicing midwifery in Washington State, many of whom had "precious little training" and currently had few opportunities to improve their skills. They were not anti-technological, but had limited access to education except for the "long, mostly irrelevant nursing-midwifery approach" that took four to five years. On top of that, there is the "large, growing community of people who are opting for childbirth at home who now have an extremely difficult time finding well trained attendants." As a result, they end up in a far riskier position of giving birth unattended or with inadequately trained midwives. Yet with a well-trained midwife, Gloyd believed birth at home might well be safer than a hospital birth.[87]

SMS would do more than simply increase the number of trained midwives, Gloyd argued; it would help to transform the very nature of health care in the United States. Since their earlier days at Fremont, the midwives had been promoting a non-hierarchical model of care that critics of modern medicine had been clamoring for. SMS would help to restore medical power to the people by "making it more possible for women, minorities, and those with fewer resources and no extensive education to become providers." Greater inclusivity and accessibility in such a program would put patient and provider on more equal footing and instill greater confidence in medicine and health.[88] Gloyd believed these midwives were the ideal people to create such a program, having themselves emerged from a similar process through the Fremont collective. After all, he had trained them.

The feedback from health professionals through letters of support undoubtedly strengthened the resulting program. In their "Proposal to Fund a Midwifery Training Program at the Seattle Midwifery School" submitted in March of 1979, SMS founders also stressed the growing need for non-nurse midwives in Washington State as well as nationwide. During their time at Fremont, they operated with a "full case load at all times," serving 300 women but turning away an equal number that they could not accommodate. By 1979, there was only one physician left in the Seattle area still offering home birth services.[89] Clearly, as Gloyd had pointed out, there was a demand for skilled attendants, as more consumers opted to give birth out of the hospital and fewer physicians were willing to serve them.

At the same time, the interest in obtaining midwifery training was on the rise. Between the time of incorporation (May 1978) and the March 1979 proposal, over 150 women had reportedly contacted SMS "from across the nation requesting to be admitted." Its founders believed this was due at least in part to the severely limited opportunities nationwide. There were only eighteen nurse-midwifery programs in the United States, and these were "exclusively hospital-birth oriented," admitting only experienced registered nurses. There were no formal schools to train non-nurse midwives, although three non-nurse groups (in Minnesota, Arizona, and Texas) offered some training. "Our intention is to fill some gaps in maternity care today by providing competent, experienced birth attendants," they declared. "There is a missing link between health care in the communities and health care in the hospitals. We hope our project will help bridge that gap."[90]

SMS founders initially developed a two-year, fourteen-month program (to comply with the vaguely worded 1917 law). In their first year, students would take didactic courses (such as anatomy and physiology), receive clinical training under the supervision of licensed clinical faculty at the Midwifery School Birth Service, and assist at home births. Their second year would be more "intensely clinical," as students would rotate through clinical training sites, spending twenty-four weeks in out-of-hospital birth services outside of the school, followed by twelve weeks at the Midwifery School Birth Service as primary midwife.[91]

THE FIRST CLASS

Perhaps the most unusual aspect of the school's beginning was the fact that the first class of students were also its founders and its board of directors.[92] They began didactic coursework for eight hours weekly in early February of 1979.[93] Initially, they had no physical space, so met in places like the Pike Place Market and Seattle Central Community College. They convinced licensed professionals to teach them free of charge (their entire initial start-up budget was $300). "We all took a Community College course in anatomy and physiology," recalls Suzy Myers. "That was really fun; I liked learning anatomy."[94] They also studied pediatrics, birth complications, embryology, and history of the family, among other subjects.[95] "Some of these are abbreviated versions, as the material is repetitious, but the instructors will formally evaluate us," they noted in the first SMS Board of Directors meeting.[96]

But what really mattered was whether the state was going to let them take the exam, since they could not be licensed without it. "That was the ultimate test, was that they allowed us to sit the licensing exam," Myers explained.[97] On January 7, 1980, Suzy Myers, Susie Rivard, Susan Anemone, Miriamma Carson, and Marge Mansfield drove to Olympia for the eight-hour exam after the required eighteen months of study. (In the meantime, they had admitted a second class of eight students, busy doing their first year of coursework.) The exam was not what they were expecting, though of course no one could predict the test format. "One question is: 'discuss gestational diabetes.' *That's* a question? And all the other questions were just like that."[98] Mansfield remembered that there were about fifteen questions.

"Discuss pre-eclampsia. Discuss diabetes. Discuss prenatal care." She was exhausted. "I just had tendonitis. I had tennis elbow, writer's cramp. All of us were just exhausted by the end of the day."[99] By the time they finished, there was a blizzard going on and they "barely made it home on I-5. It was a nightmare," according to Myers.[100]

Then the wait began. On March 25, they received the phone call: four had passed, but one had failed. "Somber afternoon," one of them wrote in their daily log. They debated asking for a second reading.[101] But in typical fashion, they didn't take it sitting down. "It was so devastating and we contested it," Suzy Myers recalls. "We said, 'oh, come on, she's the smartest one of the group. We're challenging this,'" remarked Marge. "It's just because her penmanship looks like a third-grader wrote it."[102] When they learned that they were allowed to challenge the results, they scheduled a meeting with the retired obstetrician who had written the exam and graded it. "Met Dr. Blackstone yesterday. Went over my test," noted the midwife in the daily log. "Asked to see his key for grading. He didn't have one." Together they reviewed her answers. "Went over my lowest scored essays—I still felt confident I did very well!" she wrote. "He admitted he graded too steep." When he asked her for further clarification, she provided it effectively. "You certainly do know a lot more than you wrote," he ostensibly concluded. But she didn't stop there, pushing him further to justify his grading. "When I asked if he graded on 'how' I wrote instead of 'what' I wrote he said, 'well, I'm not admitting to anything, but spelling is one of my pet peeves and maybe subconsciously it did affect your grade.' He said my answers were medically correct but 'rambely.'"[103] In the end, he accepted her challenge and changed her score to a passing grade. The showdown provided yet another example of how these midwives' persistence and determination successfully overturned established medical standards and processes.

FROM STUDENTS TO ADMINISTRATORS

As the "pilot class," the SMS founders had the opportunity to test the program out on themselves. Their next challenge was to ensure that the school could continue to successfully graduate midwifery students. Even before they were licensed, the founders had published a catalog, advertised the school, organized coursework, and admitted applicants for a second class, "all without any assurance that the program would be acceptable to the State of WA."[104] Some of the founders became the school's teachers, such as Suzy Myers, pictured in Figure 6.2. Eight students had begun coursework in the fall of 1979. Six would complete the program (one dropped

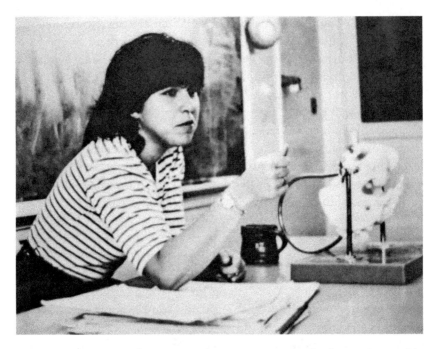

Figure 6.2 Suzy Myers teaching at SMS, ND. Suzy Myers personal collection. Reprinted by permission.

out for financial reasons, the second was dismissed due to poor academic performance).[105]

One of the new students was Teddy Charvet. By the time she attended the October 1981 ACNM meeting, she had just completed her training and had observed or managed 100 births. A month later, she passed her licensing exam and joined the SMS founders as a licensed professional midwife. Shortly after, she would become MANA's first president, drawing attention to the connections between new educational pathways (as exemplified by SMS) and professionalization (as exemplified by the founding of MANA).

Having an SMS graduate assume the presidency of MANA drew attention to the school, but it did not signify that MANA members always saw eye to eye with the SMS administrators. In 1983, for example, Suzy Myers attended the education committee meeting at the MANA convention. According to the SMS Board of Directors meeting minutes, the MANA education committee had "looked upon SMS with suspicion. They did not feel that SMS was the answer to midwifery education. Also felt that the practice of apprenticeship education needed to be preserved."[106] Though the two groups might share a passion for professionalizing non-nurse midwifery, they were far from unified in their vision of how to go about doing this.

As the creators of a new type of educational program, SMS founders found that attracting and maintaining qualified instructors proved challenging. "We regret the delay in getting the schedule of classes for the first quarter of the didactic program out to you," they wrote in their January 1981 letter to incoming students. "Several instructors were unable to teach this year and we have had difficulty replacing them."[107] Many instructors were in private practice, including nurse-midwives who were regularly called away to births at unpredictable times. This made it difficult to create a regular schedule. When students complained about particular courses or teachers, the board had little power to do anything about it, since instructors worked as adjuncts rather than tenure-track faculty.

A second challenge, also articulated in their letter to the new class of students, was legislative. For the past three years, the Washington State Midwifery Council, a group of consumers and lay midwives (including many of the SMS founders) had been working to revise the 1917 midwifery law. Among the changes they wanted to make was to create an advisory committee to assist the Department of Licensing in "promulgating standards for accrediting midwifery schools and advising the Director on issues such as continuing education and peer review." In the interest of the SMS, they wanted the revised law to "exempt students enrolled in a midwifery school and involved in supervised clinical training from the threat of being charged with illegal (unlicensed) midwifery practice."[108]

After four attempts, legislation (in the form of HB 316) was currently under consideration by the state legislature (and it would pass later that year). As the school explained to its incoming students, the bill was a product of a "diverse work group," including representatives from the Washington State Medical Association, the SMS, and the Washington State Midwifery Council. An attempt to fill in the gaps from the vaguely worded 1917 law, it included standards for midwifery training. The bill stipulated that for those students who were not registered nurses, the training period would be raised from two to three years. "Please be advised that this is proposed legislation and may not become law this year," they explained. "However, the SMS does support the passage of this bill. We feel that the standards proposed are reasonable and the establishment of such standards are vital to the future of our School and the broader acceptance of non-nurse midwifery training and practice."[109]

Not only did the incoming class of students worry about an extra year of training, they also learned that their tuition had been raised dramatically, from $1500 per year to $2500. The board was apologetic, but emphasized it was the only way the school could remain open, due to a "dangerously large deficit." While the decision to increase tuition was a difficult one, it was "necessary to the very survival of the School." As students were aware, the school was undergoing a "critical transition." The school had expanded its Board of Directors to include thirteen people as the policymaking body of the school: "It brings more energy, diversity and talent to the difficult task of steering the Midwifery School."[110]

One of those new board members was Jo Anne Myers-Ciecko. After her own home birth in 1976, she became an enthusiastic advocate of midwifery and home birth. "I felt this was something that should be available to everybody as a choice," she said. "I felt strongly about that." Her passion became organizational work around midwifery education and accreditation. "I didn't ever have a desire to be a midwife myself," she reflected, "and I suppose that if we hadn't started the school, and I hadn't been involved in this whole endeavor, I probably would have moved on to something else."[111]

Myers-Ciecko was pregnant with twins and working as a school bus driver when Suzy Myers invited her to join the SMS advisory board in 1979.[112] In 1983 she was elected executive director. "My recollection is that they knew that they needed a little more organizational framework," she said. Her role became memorialized in the Founders' Skit, when she wobbles in, hugely pregnant with twins, in between school bus shifts, attempting to run a board of directors meeting with the midwives rambling on about birth stories.[113] "It was really frustrating," she later recalled. "Because as fun as it was to hear birth stories, it wasn't what I thought was a board meeting. Then we really tried to figure out maybe hiring some staff, policies and procedures."[114] She helped to keep the group focused and on track. "It was fun for me," she said. "You know, to try to wrap my head around the puzzle of setting up an organization like this and all of the myriad details that are involved in creating a school and dealing with students, student policies, the curriculum, all that stuff, fascinating if you're trying to figure it out."[115] As an administrator, she could juggle these challenges from a more practical standpoint than the midwives.

"I NEED BIRTHS AND PLACENTAS": THE PRECEPTOR PROBLEM

Myers-Ciecko may not have been a midwife, but she knew the institutional hurdles to graduating one. Didactic coursework was only part of the training; experience was also necessary. Myers-Ciecko and the SMS found themselves in the same type of conundrum that Joseph DeLee confronted a half century earlier. Building their profession required training—in the form of hands-on experience. Yet both groups—early twentieth-century obstetricians and late-twentieth-century midwives—had limited access to birthing bodies. Both valued the benefits of training in the natural setting of the home and struggled with the decrease in available clinical material, though for very different reasons.

For DeLee, the solution had been to travel across racial and class barriers into inner-city Chicago. For midwifery educators and students, it often meant traveling across not only racial and class barriers but also geographic ones, in order to locate available subjects. "I had a taste of what is like to be in a foreign country and not speak the language," wrote Nancy Wainer Cohen during her six-week stay in 1996 at Casa de Nacimiento, a birth center located in El Paso along the Mexican border. "I just want to be here so I can do this, learn, become a midwife and be home," Cohen wrote. This was a common frustration for midwifery students desperately seeking opportunities to practice their trade. Two weeks into her stay there, Cohen became impatient at her lack of opportunity to deliver a baby. Most of her time had been spent doing prenatal exams, drawing blood, and trying to learn Spanish. "No babies," she lamented. "How will I be a midwife if there are no babies? . . . I need births and placentas."[116]

Indeed, women giving birth out of the hospital were in short supply. At the Seattle Midwifery School, each student needed to observe at least fifty births and manage, under the supervision of a licensed practitioner, another fifty in order to graduate. It was the responsibility of the school to secure preceptorships for all of their students. The most practical opportunity was the Seattle Home Maternity Service, the clinical practice of the founding members.

It quickly became evident that there were not enough births taking place through the Maternity Service to provide the necessary numbers for all students and that they would need to establish relations with outside preceptors. In February of 1980, the board decided to give prospective applicants with "pre-arranged clinical preceptors preference for admission" as one solution.[117] Even then, complications arose. The administration regularly ran into problematic situations, such as discovering after the fact that an arranged preceptor was not in fact a licensed professional, or learning that students were illegally delivering babies at home with no supervision. As founders of a new school, the last thing they needed was legal trouble.

These incidents raised larger questions about how the school could find, approve, and regulate preceptorships. "A number of students are concerned because they have submitted preceptor applications which have not yet been approved," the board noted in October of 1981. Ideally, a school representative would visit potential preceptor sites before approving them, but lack of funds made this difficult.[118] Yet the board recognized the importance of ensuring proper placement. While attending an ACNM convention in 1983, Myers was warned that SMS was "in a fishbowl" and "must be very careful to avoid slip-ups," particularly in regard to preceptorships.

A preceptor from Cincinnati apparently announced at the meeting that SMS had "abandoned" an SMS student under her watch, by failing to communicate with the student on a regular basis. SMS academic director Marge Mansfield "confirmed that while she has kept in touch with students, lack of contact with preceptors is a real problem."[119]

The real issue was not lack of contact, but a dearth of options.[120] The number of out-of-hospital births may have been increasing, but not fast enough for every student midwife to observe or participate in fifty to a hundred in a timely and affordable manner. Another option was to work with a preceptor in a hospital. But hospitals were busy training medical students, so even nurse-midwifery students such as Marion McCartney sometimes had difficulty getting their numbers. In an attempt to rectify the situation, Mansfield proposed that students should manage thirty, rather than fifty births over the course of their training. As a way to increasing oversight, she also offered to meet with each student on a regular basis to track the number of births attended. If students were still having trouble getting enough opportunities, perhaps a preceptorship abroad would be possible.[121]

ST. LUCIA AND THE PROBLEM
OF MIDWIFERY TOURISM

By January of 1982, Mansfield had done more research on the possibilities of foreign preceptorships, where restrictions against non-nurse midwives was less common. She noted that eight SMS students were planning on rotating through St. Jude's hospital in St. Lucia, and one planned to work in Brazil. Some members of the SMS education committee expressed concern about different standards of care in foreign countries, suggesting that the school "reassess this policy periodically."[122]

The problem went far deeper than simply "different standards of care." What the education committee and SMS more generally failed to address until decades later was the questionable ethics of out-of-country midwifery training. This was not just an issue for the SMS; sociologist Sheryl Nestel recently discovered that a large number of midwives in Ontario had "garnered the requisite quota of births" in Third World maternity clinics.[123] Nestel describes this process as a form of "midwifery tourism," a process that has made pregnant Third World bodies "available for the educational consumption and material advantage of First World women."[124]

By applying the discourse of "global sisterhood," midwifery students (primarily white and middle class) deflected ethical questions of race and imperialism. Midwife and educator Wendy Gordon, who graduated from SMS in 2005, later articulated how this discourse enabled her to avoid deeper questions of race, privilege, and power while training in a developing country. "I didn't think much about these power dynamics, because I convinced myself that the gentle, woman-centered type of care I was trained to provide would benefit all mothers and babies, even across international boundaries and language barriers," she reflected.[125]

But in the 1980s, the implications of midwifery tourism were not discussed, at least not among midwifery students or program administrators. The promise that such preceptorships offered to the burgeoning practice of non-nurse midwifery effectively prevented dissent. An examination of the SMS/St. Lucia preceptorships at St. Jude's and Victoria Hospital, however, reveals the ways in which on-the-ground experiences, assumptions, and miscommunications began to fracture the myth of global sisterhood.

By 1986, twenty-five SMS students had completed six- to eight-week rotations at St. Jude's hospital in St. Lucia, a country with 142,000 inhabitants, 60 percent of whom were "functionally illiterate."[126] St. Jude's was a Catholic hospital that opened in 1966 with funds raised by Sister Mary Irma Hilger and her religious order, the Sisters of the Sorrowful Mother, from Oshkosh, Wisconsin. Hilger had come to St. Lucia to work as a nurse at Victoria Hospital, the island's main hospital, in 1960, where she started the first nursing school on the island. After being approached by local Catholics interested in starting a Catholic hospital, she began her mission to establish one at the southern tip of the island, in Vieux Fort.[127] By 1987, the 107-bed hospital served approximately 60,000 people.[128]

Signs of problems with the St. Jude's preceptorship started as early as 1983, when hospital administrator Sr. Sharee expressed "concerns and frustrations" with SMS students, who were not meeting her expectations.[129] Mansfield responded in July, but the letter was delayed. One of the SMS students in St. Lucia at the time wrote Mansfield to relay Sr. Sharee's "further frustration" at not having received any response from the school. Another student who had recently returned also relayed messages of Sr. Sharee's "discomfiture." Mansfield agreed to phone and "reiterate the contents of the as yet unreceived letter," including their desire to "confirm/comply with Sr. Sharee's expectations."[130] But perhaps it was too little too late, making the possibility for reconciliation all the less likely.

A few months later, Sr. Sharee made it clear in a telephone call that in order for the preceptorship to continue, certain changes would have to take place that would alter the balance of power. First, she explained, St. Jude's would no longer offer a stipend to SMS students or provide free room and board. Undoubtedly the hospital had very limited funds; she probably realized they could be better spent on St. Lucia residents than presumably wealthy Americans. This decision was perhaps an indication that the clinical rotation in her hospital benefited SMS students more than the patients or hospital staff. Second, Sr. Sharee asked that future student groups be accompanied by a tutor, someone with a nursing degree and one to two years of experience outside of midwifery school. She may have felt that SMS students were requiring too much time and training by her own staff.

Her second request would prove the undoing of the St. Jude's preceptorship. SMS could not provide a tutor with the qualifications of a nursing degree to accompany their students.[131] This request drew attention to the fault lines in the very foundation of the St. Lucia preceptorship agreement. If the student midwives proved incapable of working at St. Jude's without an SMS-provided tutor, perhaps they should not be there in the first place. At a meeting of the SMS Steering Committee, faculty and administrators expressed concern about the "relative inexperience" of the students they were sending to St. Lucia "(some coming almost directly from the didactic part of the program)."[132] Perhaps it was time to reassess the wisdom of out-of-country rotations.

Instead of terminating international preceptorships, SMS sought to refine them. By 1986, Mansfield had established relations with the main health care facility, Victoria Hospital, which appeared more willing to work with the school. When approaching the head nurse at Victoria, Mansfield was careful to articulate her expectations from the start in the hopes of avoiding another conflict. "Did I understand you correctly in saying accommodations including board could be provided there at the Hospital?" she asked. "Would there be a charge for room and/or board?" Then she proceeded with her main concern—the role and definition of the preceptor. "Would each student work specifically under the supervision of one or two staff midwives?" she asked. "Would one be designated as the official preceptor, responsible as a liaison, for orientation and evaluation?"[133] Receiving a favorable reply, she made arrangements for two students to start the following summer.

The century-old hospital stood on a nine-acre site overlooking the capital city of Castries and offered breathtaking views of the Caribbean ocean.[134] Roughly half of St. Lucia's fifty-five physicians practiced at the 211-bed hospital in the mid-1980s. Only eight of them were locals; the rest had been recruited from abroad, especially from South Asia.[135] Between April of 1986 and March of 1987, 2,284 babies were born at the hospital, 129 by cesarean section (representing a rate of 5.6 percent, dramatically lower than the U.S. rate of 24 percent that year).[136]

The new arrangement in St. Lucia appealed to incoming SMS students, whose postcards home detailed the excitement and adventure of midwifery tourism and the sheer beauty of the hospital site overlooking the Caribbean ocean. "This is the most amazing experience!" wrote an SMS student to her classmates in Seattle in June of 1987. Travel to a developing country was completely foreign to them. "Our arrival was such an incredibly disastrous culture shock, I thought we'd never recover, let alone adjust. But, after a little more than a week, we're beginning to." She described their rooms as "10x10 concrete with light green dirty walls, water stained ceilings, holes rotted in the floor big enough for a rat (although we haven't seen any yet)." Chickens, goats, sheep, dogs and cats roamed through the hospital grounds. The hospital made her nauseous the first day but she had grown to like it. It consisted of two rooms connected by a nurse's station the size of a desk. Twenty-eight beds filled the rooms, and the hospital had been full since she had arrived there.[137]

Another student who arrived a few months later echoed her classmate's enthusiasm for St. Lucia. Her postcard was sprinkled with various observations that alluded to its appeal as a tourist destination. "It's heaven," she wrote from her perch on a rock on "the most beautiful beach ever." She perceived the laid-back attitude of the island's inhabitants as refreshingly different from the frenetic pace of Americans. "The favorite saying of the locals is 'no problem' and that is how they take life," she wrote enthusiastically. This mindset, she believed, shaped hospital practices as well. "The hospital experience here has really opened my mind to relax after my experiences of paranoia in the U.S. hospitals."[138] The interventionist techniques so often practiced in American maternity wards appeared to have no place in such a culture, although, as she points out, they lacked basic supplies; even stethoscopes were in "short supply." Perhaps the laid-back approach she observed stemmed from resignation and resilience in the face of poverty, rather than a "happy-go-lucky" mentality.

She then quickly contradicted this observation by vilifying the local midwives, whom she found to be anything but laid back. "The hardest part of our experience has been accepting the attitude and manners of the St. Lucian midwives," she wrote. They did not appear to exhibit any of the nurturing or supportive traits that she associated with midwifery. "There is a certain hardness in dealing with the laboring women that is so different from the SMS midwifery approach," she explained. Any notion of a "global sisterhood" of midwives would have been quickly crushed by her observations.

Other SMS student midwives spoke of the ambivalence and confusion they felt while witnessing the interaction between local midwives and laboring women in St. Lucia. "The midwives would yell at the mothers," remembered Beth Coyote, who was there in the mid-1980s. "They'd slap women," she explained. "Just even the tiniest amount of tenderness was frowned upon." Her classmate was horrified, but Coyote tried to keep an open mind and "learned not to make value judgments." Neither of them expected births in St. Lucia to be characterized by physical violence.[139]

In 1992, two SMS student midwives who rotated through Victoria Hospital were so taken aback by hospital practices that they decided to write a five-page "survival guide" for future midwifery students. Karen Hays and Sarah Huntington were even more disturbed by what they saw than the postcard writers from earlier years. "Be emotionally prepared to stand by while the laboring woman suffers lots of verbal abuse and unconsented upon procedures which are painful," they wrote. They viewed the local midwife/patient relationship as extremely hierarchical. "For some reason the midwives feel compelled to establish some severe power differential between themselves and the patients, and try to motivate the patients with threats."[140] In her study of Canadian midwives who acquired the requisite number of births in developing countries, Nestel found a similar reaction. Many described feeling "profoundly disturbed by the lack of respect and absence of choice that characterized the care in which they participated."[141]

Perhaps even more disturbing to the SMS students was when they found themselves implicated in interactions or procedures that they assumed were not in the laboring mother's best interest. These procedures challenged their assumptions about island midwifery. There was nothing "natural" about it; instead, it appeared to replicate the Western medical model SMS midwives were attempting to replace. "You will get proficient at giving soap suds enemas, and shaving pubic hair. I tried to avoid that for a while, but eventually I had to do this," wrote one student in 1986. She also noted that mediolateral episiotomies, such as the one Suzy Myers complained about during her own labor, were "preferred and frequent." [142] The two 1992 authors of the "survival guide" warned of the need to be "psychologically and emotionally prepared for not being able to control what happens to your patient." Their warning revealed the contestations for power between the students and local midwives. "You may feel like you've 'claimed' a patient by doing her admit etc., but the midwives will generally start an IV or Foley cath[eter] or give Pain meds without consulting you or even over your objections," they wrote.[143] In this narrative, the patient becomes a commodity of whom both groups claim ownership. Student midwives, present only for brief stints, resisted the notion that as outsiders they did not have the right to assert control. Local midwives undoubtedly viewed these white privileged American students more as a hindrance than a help.

Yet as the very term *survival guide* suggests, the primary intention of the student midwives was to fill a quota. As student midwife Nancy Wainer Cohen had written, "I need births and placentas." They just had to get by. Navigating hospital politics and understanding staff hierarchies was half the battle. "The staff is cordial, but standoffish at first," observed students Hays and Huntington. "Win them over midwife by midwife. Sister Paul is definitely unfriendly; don't take it personally," they noted. "Be ready to deal with lots of criticism; almost everything you do is wrong, and you have to do things their way. You'll know you did something right by the fact that they didn't tell you you did it wrong (i.e. they'll be silent)." [144] The most important thing to bring, they advised, was "your most cherished inspirational midwifery/birthing book," which would help you "stay focused in the midst of their version of the <u>medical</u> model!"[145] The key was to get the requisite number of births completed in order to graduate.

Perhaps because of her own experiences abroad, "survival guide" author Karen Hays developed a questionnaire for SMS graduates on their experiences in foreign training sites. Why had they chosen out-of-country preceptorships? Fifty-nine graduates responded, all of whom had worked in a developing country for an average of three to eight weeks. The most frequently cited answer was "achieving the number of births required for graduation." Other answers included an interest in the cross-cultural experience, an opportunity to improve clinical skills, a taste for adventure, and "an interest in seeing obstetrical complications." As SMS graduate Lisa Delorme later argued, none of the justifications involved an interest in benefiting the host community. She viewed these answers as "a clear demonstration of the unilateral and unequal exchange that is a major ethical issue inherent in many international clinical rotations."[146]

Delorme's findings were part of a wider examination of overseas preceptor sites in the midwifery community in the twenty-first century. They helped to raise awareness of the downside of international preceptorships like those in St. Lucia and, ultimately, contributed to the school's decision to terminate the "longstanding tradition" of international preceptorships in September of 2013. "Over the years questions and concerns have been raised about whether the School should take more responsibility for adequate preparation of students and oversight of their experiences while 'in country,'" administrators wrote. But after another American training program, Midwife International, was called to task for unethical behavior and exploitation in its use of clinical sites in developing countries, administrators believed it was "time to take stock of our own house."[147] Questions were to be directed to Suzy Myers as department chair.

AFTER GRADUATION

Initially, some SMS graduates struggled to develop a practice after obtaining their certificate. One of the members of the second class set up a practice on the east side of Seattle just after graduating. "She has invested a great deal in publicity but as yet has no clients," noted one of the SMS administrators after speaking with her. The graduate suggested that SMS should think about developing alumni networks and work on generating more publicity for the school "among medical people." She noted how challenging it was to establish a working partnership with a doctor, "to face the blank stares when she told them where she had gone to school. None of them had heard of the SMS," she explained. She also suggested that SMS offer more "how to" courses as part of their curriculum, "particularly on how to approach banks for loans, setting up a bookkeeping system, etc."[148]

Beth Coyote, who has been practicing midwifery in Seattle since graduating from SMS in 1986, believes that SMS gave her a "good foundation" to be a successful midwife. The combination of didactic coursework and preceptorships provided her with the right balance of training and experience. She continues to serve as a preceptor to midwifery students through her Seattle practice, Rainy City Midwifery. "My current student is in clinic with us all the time," she noted in 2015. "Just she's either in clinic or she's at births and she's constantly absorbing." Among other things, preceptorships were important "because so much of what we're imparting to students is the subtleties. How do you read somebody's body language when they're sitting in front of you?" Yet she also found the curriculum provided in a "classroom environment where there's a teacher and there's other students to talk things through, I mean I think that that's one of the values of an education like [SMS]."[149] Indeed, in a 1985 "Politics of Health Care" class taught by Jo Anne Myers-Ciecko and Marcia Peterson, Coyote actively participated in a discussion over the benefits and drawbacks of partnering with doctors. Her active engagement suggests the extent to which she valued and benefited from classroom discussion.[150]

Coyote represented a new type of SMS student in the mid-1980s: those coming from out of state. She had been involved in home birth in Syracuse before heading out to the West Coast, and relocated to Seattle when she learned about the school. Myers-Ciecko spoke of the shift in the student body. "When the school first opened, our students mostly came from Washington State," she noted. "Most of them had had significant midwifery experience prior to enrolling." As word of the school got out, more students traveled to enroll. Some of them had prior midwifery experience, but many did not. By 1997, SMS students ranged in age from twenty-one to sixty-five, but were typically women in their thirties and early forties. They were overwhelmingly white, though there were three African-American women students that year. "We are really excited about them, because they have such a passion for re-connecting midwifery to their communities," Myers-Ciecko stated. Gradually, the school began the difficult discussions and strategies surrounding diversity, which would lead them to the 2013 decision to work to "dismantle racism in midwifery education" by suspending the preceptorships in developing countries.[151]

By 2002, 185 students had graduated from SMS, forty-nine of whom were listed as living out of state in the 2002 alumni directory. Graduates were offering midwifery services in Canada, California, Oregon, Montana, Colorado, Michigan, Wisconsin, Illinois, Ohio, Arizona, Hawaii, Maine, New Mexico, Alaska, Rhode Island, Virginia, and Vermont. They had opened practices such as "Ruby Slippers Midwifery" in Homer, Alaska, and "LifeJoy Midwifery" in Kelowna, British Columbia.[152] As a nationally accredited institution (and indeed, administrator Myers-Ciecko became a founding member of MEAC, the agency developed to offer a national accreditation program to non-nurse midwifery schools), the Seattle Midwifery School played a major role in transforming non-nurse midwifery into an established profession in the United States.

In the spring of 2010, SMS founders Marge Mansfield and Suzy Myers spoke at the graduation of the thirtieth class of the Seattle Midwifery School. It was to be the last class of SMS, which had completed a merger with Bastyr University in 2009. In lieu of performing their traditional skit of the school's founding, they showed PowerPoint slides. Photographs of the early days— the original group posing in front of the Fremont Women's Clinic, the influential books such as Ina May Gaskin's *Spiritual Midwifery* and Raven Lang's *Birth Book*, portraits of doctors Tom Artzner and Steve Gloyd, and of course, Roz Woodhouse, the Director of Licensing—punctuated the quips and memories of their thirty-year history.

As with many commencement addresses, this one ended with hopes for the future. "It has definitely 'taken a village' to get here," noted Mansfield, "and now that we've told you about the legacy we're leaving you, we get to tell you what to do with your lives, right? We want you, our successors to serve women and catch babies by partnering with clients and colleagues, building community, socially, non-hierarchically; working with one or more midwives, supporting each other and exemplifying a healthy lifestyle in which you have integrity, balance, and longevity."[153]

Myers chimed in, noting that after forty years as a practicing midwife, she was "too old to get up in the middle of the night" and therefore appreciating her role as a teacher more than ever. "Maybe someday, you'll consider trading your pager for a course syllabus," she told the graduates. "All along we've been true to our mission to educate and inspire leaders. It has been my great pleasure to see students become colleagues and graduates become leaders. I expect nothing less of you! Get involved, be activist midwives, be the change you want to see in your world," she exhorted.[154] Looking out at the young, hopeful faces of the class of 2010, she undoubtedly remembered when she first set out to both become a licensed midwife and to start a school. She mentioned in 2015 that she believes that there was this "little

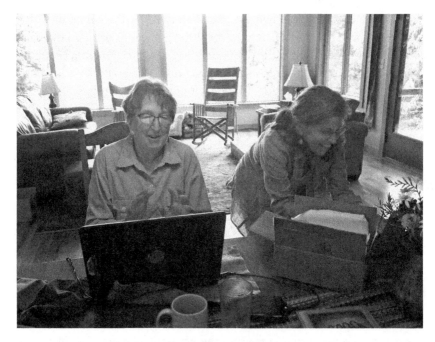

Figure 6.3 Jo Anne Myers-Ciecko and Suzy Myers perusing historic SMS documents, in Myers-Ciecko home, July 22, 2015. Photograph by Wendy Kline. Reprinted by permission.

dose of magic" that enabled all the pieces to fall into place that created the Seattle Midwifery School.[155] But it was largely due to the determination and commitment of a handful of women and men who were willing to risk their futures on the idea that midwifery education was the key to professionalization.

It was not an easy challenge. The founders were young women when they came together in the mid-1970s, and as they matured along with the school, they faced both philosophical and practical hurdles. Initially, they embraced their position as anti-establishment outsiders who were opposed to licensure. But their growing recognition that they needed to establish working relationships with hospital staff forced them to rethink this position. Incorporating the school, developing a curriculum, hiring faculty, and training students required a level of professionalism that their earlier selves might have snubbed. In addition, the "preceptor problem" forced them to come to terms with their ethically debatable overseas programs—even if it appeared to be a practical way of attaining the requisite number of births at a time when it was difficult to do so at home. As is often the case with educational reform, institutional change sometimes required the demands of students rather than the administration. In 2006, for example, SMS student leaders organized to address racism in midwifery education, and as a result, anti-racism training became a school-wide requirement.[156]

The merger with Bastyr University signaled a new chapter in the history of the Seattle Midwifery School, bringing together two thirty-year-old institutions centered on health care. Bastyr opened in 1978 as a college of naturopathic medicine. In 2007 the two schools began discussing a proposed affiliation, hopeful that a merger would expand midwifery education offerings and enable SMS to transform its midwifery certificate program into a regionally accredited degree program. Offering a degree program for midwifery students "has long been a part of our strategic plan," explained Mary Yglesia, executive director of SMS in 2009. "It has not been achievable as a small, independent school, and by joining resources with a much larger regionally accredited institution we can reach this goal." The new Department of Midwifery launched in 2009, and currently has twenty-four faculty members and offers two master's degree programs: A Master of Arts in Maternal-Child Health Systems, and a Master of Science in Midwifery.[157] What had started as an experimental program held in coffee shops and community centers had finally settled on a beautiful 186,000-square-foot campus surrounded by fifty-one acres of fields and woodlands.

Epilogue

In Search of Common Ground

For three days in September 2014, ninety-three delegates participated in the third Home Birth Summit at the "discreet, quintessentially Northwest hideaway" Cedarbrook Lodge outside of Seattle, Washington.[1] Nurse-midwives, direct-entry midwives, obstetricians, general practitioners, nurses, activists, philosophers, historians, epidemiologists, activists, a documentary film maker, and representatives from ACNM, MANA, and ACOG wrangled with the current policies, regulation, evidence, and ethics of home birth in the United States. "We are in a time of rapid change in the discourse on health care, access, and disparities in the United States," explained Saraswathi Vedam, Associate Professor of Midwifery at the University of British Columbia and chair of the Home Birth Summit Steering Council. "This is an ideal opportunity to consult with each other as we address challenging topics, including the ethics of birth place decision-making, inter-professional conflict and collaboration, risk management, consumer directed research projects, as well as the mandates for increased safety, equity, access, consumer engagement, and physiologic birth care."[2] Heated discussions took place in meeting rooms, but conviviality and collaboration increased over after-dinner drinks and outdoor strolls. Regardless of individual stakeholder's perspectives, the shared passion for improving maternal and infant health outcomes was potent.

Vedam was not exaggerating regarding the rapidly changing discourse on health care in the United States, currently the most expensive place in the world to give birth.[3] Despite this, birth is far from safe. Severe maternal complications have doubled over the last twenty years.[4] America's maternal mortality rate is currently worse than it was twenty-five years ago—a distinction only thirteen countries in the world hold.[5] In addition, the United States has a higher infant mortality rate than any of the other wealthy countries, according to a CDC report, a statistic condemned by the *Washington Post* as a "national embarrassment."[6]

The purpose of the third and final Home Birth Summit was to formalize action plans based on "common ground principles" that had been developed in the 2011 and 2013 summits. While it was clear that no formal consensus could be reached regarding the future of home birth, delegates came up with ten "common ground statements" intended to encourage "dialogue and collaboration across sectors" in order to work toward a "common goal of improving maternal and newborn care for families choosing home birth."[7]

The desire for collaboration was widespread. "We believe that collaboration within an integrated maternity care system is essential for optimal mother–baby outcomes," delegates wrote at the 2011 meeting. "When ongoing inter-professional dialogue and cooperation occur, everyone benefits."[8] Collaboration was also extremely challenging, given the "historically opposing views" that prevented improving the integration of maternity care services for all women and families. "Is Home Birth Ever a Safe Choice?" asked the *New York Times* in a 2015 discussion forum. It depended on who you asked. "A hospital or birthing center continues to be the safest place for labor and delivery," stressed the president of ACOG; "evidence shows that although the overall risk of serious childbirth complications remains low, there is still a twofold to threefold increased risk of neonatal death associated with home birth."[9] The president of MANA disagreed, pointing to a "growing body of research" that demonstrates that "for women with low-risk pregnancies and access to medical back-up if needed, home birth with a skilled provider is a safe option."[10]

The problem, according to ACOG, was a lack of high-quality evidence. "To date, there have been no adequate randomized clinical trials of planned home birth," the organization stated in 2017. Most published studies were observational and therefore "limited by methodological problems" such as small sample sizes, lack of a control group, and reliance on voluntary submission of data.[11]

Stakeholders at the third Home Birth Summit shared a similar concern over the lack of data. "To date, there are no high quality population-based, prospective, cohort studies in the United States that compare outcomes across birth settings," Vedam explained. On the second day of the summit, she led a half-day US Birth Place Study Planning Meeting, designed to convene a research team consisting of experts across maternity care professions "because of the significant divergence in accepting the credibility of studies on home birth."[12] She hoped that the meeting would galvanize interested experts to identify key research questions, data sources, and methods. A well-researched, accurate study could have a major impact on the future of home birth practices.

Jessica Moore, a family nurse practitioner, agreed. She attended the 2014 summit in search of evidence and to interview Vedam for her first documentary film, *Why Not Home? The Surprising Choices of Doctors and Nurses*. The mother of two young children born at home, she worked in a health center where two of her colleagues, an obstetrician and a nurse, had also chosen to give birth at home. "These are not the women most Americans picture when they imagine a home birth mom," Moore explains of herself and her colleagues.[13] As health professionals trained in hospital settings, they found themselves "in the firing line for some pretty harsh personal and professional criticism."[14] Moore set out to "face homebirth data head on" in search of answers, not just anecdotal evidence. "I need to speak to some experts. People who could help me separate the evidence from all the noise out there." [15]

She was not disappointed. "It was encouraging to see people with varied backgrounds work through their differences and come to some consensus on things like home to hospital transfers," she reflected. She selected film footage of the Home Birth Summit that effectively conveyed the respectful but intense debates about how to move forward. The room grew silent, for example, when British-trained midwife and women's health advocate Jennie Joseph spoke up during a session on "the ethics of home birth and informed decision-making." The most challenging problem the United States faced, Joseph argued, was access to prenatal care. "We have to acknowledge that prenatal care in the United States of America is not a human right. Right now. We have to acknowledge that you can't just up and get prenatal care."[16] Joseph was speaking from experience; as the owner of The Birth Place birthing center in Florida, the majority of her clients are low-income African Americans, Haitians, and Latinas. She will not turn away a patient "regardless of ability to pay or health insurance status."[17] Most of them have nowhere else to go. She views her support staff—from the receptionist to medical assistants to educators—as "critical parts of the team that help mothers get to term safely." The results are impressive; preterm birth and low-infant birth weight rates among her clients are "significantly lower than rates in other settings."[18]

Summit delegates agreed that this sort of teamwork is lacking in the U.S. healthcare system. Vedam, who spent twenty-five years working as a midwife in the United States before moving to British Columbia, noted the difference in cultural practices. In British Columbia, home birth is integrated into the health care system, whereas in the United States it is entirely separate. "If every time you have a normal birth at home the entire system is aware, it changes the idea of what planned home birth is about . . . when you have an integrated system, everybody benefits," Vedam explained to Moore.[19]

In February of 2018, Vedam successfully provided scientific evidence to support this claim. "Mapping integration of midwives across the United States: Impact on access, equity, and outcomes" was published in the peer-reviewed journal *PLOS One.* Vedam and her coauthors noted that despite studies demonstrating the benefits of midwifery care, access to such care is "markedly lower" than in most other countries. Midwives attend approximately 10 percent of all U.S. births compared to 50–75 percent in other "high-resource countries." Furthermore, not all of them are integrated into regional health care systems. "American midwives face multiple challenges to practice, including numerous regulatory barriers and inability to secure third party reimbursement," they argue.[20]

As a result, many women do not have access to midwifery care. This, in turn, limits birthplace options, as most home and birth center births are presided over by a midwife. "Choice of birth place is functionally quite limited for a majority of U.S. women," the authors point out. Their groundbreaking study offers the first systematic and comprehensive investigation of state regulations for midwifery practice, and their findings are telling. States that have integrated midwifery care into their health care systems have better birth outcomes than states that have not. They developed a model for ranking states, which they call the Midwifery Integration Scoring System, suggesting that it can help to identify those states where women and children "might benefit from improved integration of midwives." State scores ranged from a low of 17 (North Carolina) to a high of 61 (Washington state). Those states with a higher density of midwives and a higher proportion of midwife-attended births also had lower rates of cesarean section, low-birth-weight infants, and neonatal mortality.[21]

Their findings suggest that greater integration of midwives into the health care system can also reduce health disparities. "Density of midwives and access to midwives across birth settings were also significantly lower in states where more black babies are born," they explain.[22] Studies have shown that African-American women experience two to four times higher risk than white women for maternal and infant mortality. A middle-class African-American woman with an advanced degree was "more likely to lose her baby than a white woman with less than an eighth-grade education," new studies show.[23] The findings are far more grim in particular areas; in New York City, African-American women are twelve times more likely to die from childbirth complications than white women.[24] These statistics have generated headlines such as that on the cover of the April 11, 2018 *New York Times Magazine*: "Why America's Black Mothers and Babies Are in a Life-or-Death Crisis." The fact that Vedam's recent study offers a potential solution to racial disparities in birth outcomes makes it all the more relevant.

Among those who have praised this study is obstetrician Neel Shah, assistant professor at Harvard Medical School. Alarmed at the high rates of cesarean sections nationwide and the lack of maternity care in particular regions, he supports integrating midwifery care more fully into the health care system. "Growing our workforce, including both midwives and obstetricians, and then ensuring we have a regulatory environment that facilitates integrated, team-based care are key parts of the solution," he believes.[25]

What is missing in twenty-first-century reports of the current status of midwifery, birthplace options, and birth outcomes is an awareness of the earlier collaborative efforts between some doctors, midwives, and consumers. Despite competition, criticism, and crises, attempts to improve the birthing experience started well before the year 2000. Many individuals and organizations confronted legislative, professional, and educational hurdles, determined to make birth both safe and meaningful for everyone involved.

Twenty-first century medicine thrives on scientific evidence to ensure best practices. But questions about what evidence to include and how to interpret it invariably polarize different patients and practitioners. "Is home birth ever safe?" asked the *New York Times* in 2015. Is it selfish or responsible for a laboring mother to opt out of the hospital? These questions have been asked repeatedly, without true engagement or awareness of the historical framework from which these debates originated. Unless Dr. Joseph DeLee's statements on the safety of home birth are included alongside his denigration of midwives, or the link between home birth doctors and midwives and the Chicago Maternity Center is acknowledged, we are left with a distorted view of how modern midwifery and home birth coalesced in the mid-twentieth century. Without the stories of middle-class suburban leaders of home birth advocacy groups, we lack the ability to recognize who was involved in the movement and why. When Lester Hazell conducted an ethnographic study of 300 home births in California from 1969–1973 for her Master's thesis, she uncovered something surprising. "Contrary to usual assumption, people electing to have home births in the San Francisco Bay Area appear to be quite average," she concluded. Ninety percent of them "lived in stereotyped American fashion—single family dwelling, fathers gainfully employed," and not on welfare.[26] Jessica Moore, the filmmaker who attended the Home Birth Summit to learn more about current practices, wanted to demonstrate in her documentary that a typical "home birth mom" could be, well, anyone.

The same was true forty years earlier. It was the art student in San Francisco, the nurse in Santa Cruz, the La Leche League leader in Takoma Park, the community activist in Seattle, and the hippie midwife on The Farm. Collectively, they educated themselves, published newsletters and books, collaborated with physicians and psychiatrists, challenged legal restrictions, taught childbirth education classes, created professional organizations, and developed educational guidelines. They faced challenges along the way, both from within their own groups and from those opposed to what they were doing. But they helped to shape the movement that remains with us today, one that is now increasingly diverse and politically savvy. The movement, in turn, has enabled parents to navigate an increasingly complex health care system in order to make well-informed choices about where and how to give birth. Yet most Americans have no idea how unique or arduous the path has been that brought us where we are today.

NOTES

INTRODUCTION

1. http://abcnews.go.com/Health/Wellness/gisele-bundchen-makes-water-births-sexy-delivering-son/story?id=9721599.
2. https://www.popsugar.com/moms/Celebrities-Who-Have-Chosen-Home-Births-17988403.
3. http://abcnews.go.com/Health/Wellness/gisele-bundchen-makes-water-births-sexy-delivering-son/story?id=9721599.
4. Mairi Breen Rothman, CNM, MSN, Public Health Practice Grand Rounds, MidAtlantic Public Health Training Center, Johns Hopkins University, July 20, 2011.
5. Robbie Davis-Floyd, quoted in http://www.sandiegouniontribune.com/sdut-home-birth-on-the-rise-by-a-dramatic-20-percent-2011jul05-story.html.
6. Richard W. Wertz and Dorothy C. Wertz, *Lying-In: A History of Childbirth in America* (New York: Free Press, 1977), 1.
7. Judith Walzer Leavitt, *Brought to Bed: Childbearing in America, 1750–1950* (New York: Oxford University Press, 1986), 36.
8. Ibid., 38–39.
9. Ibid., 39.
10. Ballard quoted in Laurel Thatcher Ulrich, *A Midwife's Tale: The Life of Martha Ballard, Based on her Diary, 1784–1812* (New York: Knopf, 1990), 177.
11. Leavitt, *Brought to Bed*, 57.
12. Charlotte Borst, *Catching Babies: The Professionalization of Childbirth, 1870–1920* (Cambridge: Harvard University Press, 1995), 1.
13. Patricia Cloyd Carter, *Come Gently, Sweet Lucina* (Titusville, FL: Patricia Cloyd Carter, 1957), 292.
14. Pamela E. Klassen, *Blessed Events: Religion and Home Birth in America* (Princeton: Princeton University Press, 2001), 29.
15. Carter, *Come Gently, Sweet Lucina*, 337.
16. Linda S. quoted in Dorothy Cupich, "Special Deliveries: There's a Revolution Going on in Childbirth," *Philadelphia Magazine* [n.d.].
17. Dorothy Cupich, "Special Deliveries: There's a Revolution Going on in Childbirth," *Philadelphia Magazine*, p. 184.
18. William C. Scott, "Lay Midwives: Some Solutions to a Serious Problem," *Contemporary Ob/Gyn* Vol. 16, September 1980, p. 37.
19. Barbara Katz Rothman, *In Labor: Women and Power in the Birthplace* (New York: Norton, 1991) p. 15.

20. Judy Norsigian and Jane Pincus, "Preface," in Sagov, Feinbloom, Spindel, and Brodsky, editors, *Home Birth: A Practitioner's Guide to Birth outside the Hospital* (Rockville: Aspen Systems Corporation, 1984), p. xv.

21. For more on the history of childbirth, see Charlotte Borst, *Catching Babies: The Professionalization of Childbirth, 1870–1920* (Cambridge: Harvard University Press, 1995); Robbie Davis-Floyd, *Birth as an American Rite of Passage* (Berkeley: University of California Press, 1992); Raymond DeVries, *Making Midwives Legal: Childbirth, Medicine, and the Law* (Columbus: Ohio State University Press, 1996); Klassen, *Blessed Events: Religion and Home Birth in America* (Princeton: Princeton University Press, 2001); Judith Walzer Leavitt, *Brought to Bed: Childbearing in America, 1750-1950* (New York: Oxford University Press, 1986, 2016); Judith Walzer Leavitt, *Make Room for Daddy: The Journey from Waiting Room to Birthing Room* (Chapel Hill: University of North Carolina Press, 2010); Paula Michaels, *Lamaze: An International History* (New York: Oxford University Press, 2014); Judith Rooks, *Midwifery and Childbirth in America* (Philadelphia: Temple University Press, 1999); Julia Chinyere Oparah and Alicia D. Bonaparte, eds., *Birthing Justice: Black Women, Pregnancy, and Childbirth* (New York: Routledge, 2016); Barbara Katz Rothman, *In Labor: Women and Power in the Birthplace* (New York: Norton, 1991); Richard W. Wertz and Dorothy C. Wertz, *Lying-In: A History of Childbirth in America* (New York: Free Press, 1977); Jacqueline Wolf, *Cesarean Section: An American History of Risk, Technology, and Consequence* (Baltimore: Johns Hopkins University Press, 2018).

22. Richard Horton and Olaya Asutdillo, "The Power of Midwifery," *The Lancet*, Vol. 384 Issue 9948, (Sept. 20, 2014): 1075–1076.

23. "International Day of the Midwife 2018: A Message from MANA President Vicki Hedley," *MANA* Newsletter, Issue #75, May 4, 2018.

CHAPTER 1

1. Kay Furey interview with author June 2015, Chicago, IL.

2. Both of these have been the subject of historical inquiry; yet existing historical accounts do not position their histories within the wider context of the home birth movement. See Lynn Weiner, "Reconstructing Motherhood: The La Leche League in Postwar America," *The Journal of American History* 80(4) (1994): 1357–1381; Carolyn Herbst Lewis, "The Gospel of Good Obstetrics: Joseph Bolivar DeLee's Vision for Childbirth in the United States," *Social History of Medicine* 29(1) (2016): 112–130.

3. See Jacqueline H. Wolf, *Deliver Me from Pain: Anesthesia and Birth in America* (Baltimore: Johns Hopkins University Press, 2009), p. 84; Lewis, "The Gospel of Good Obstetrics," 112–130.

4. Judith Leavitt, "Joseph DeLee and the Practice of Preventive Obstetrics," *American Journal of Public Health* 78(10)(1988): 1353.

5. Constance D. Leupp and Marguerite Tracy, "Childbirth: Nature v. Drugs," *Time*, Vol. 27, Issue 21, May 25, 1936.

6. Morris Fishbein, in conjunction with Sol Theron DeLee, *Joseph Bolivar DeLee: Crusading Obstetrician* (Boston: Dutton, 1949), 11.

7. Ibid., p. 110.

8. Charlotte Borst, *Catching Babies: The Professionalization of Childbirth* (Harvard University Press, 1995), p. 97.

9. Quoted in Fishbein, *Crusading Obstetrician*, 46.

10. Charles E. Rosenberg, *The Care of Strangers: The Rise of America's Hospital System* (Baltimore: Johns Hopkins University Press, 1995), p. 170.

11. DeLee, 1938, quoted in Fishbein, *Crusading Obstetrician*, 46–47.

12. Judith Walzer Leavitt, *Brought to Bed: Childbearing in America, 1750–1950* (Oxford University Press 1988), p. 59.
13. Fishbein, *Crusading Obstetrician*, 49. For more on the New York Dispensary, see Nancy Schrom Dye, "Modern Obstetrics and Working-Class Women: The New York Midwifery Dispensary, 1890–1920," *Journal of Social History* 20(3) (Spring 1987): 549–564.
14. Joseph B. DeLee, *Chicago Lying-in Hospital—First Annual Report* (Chicago: 1895–96), 6.
15. Fishbein, *Crusading Obstetrician*, 51.
16. DeLee, *First Annual Report*, 6.
17. Ibid., 8.
18. This was the decade when "women in alliance with obstetrical specialists decided to move childbirth to the hospital," as Judith Leavitt describes in *Brought to Bed*, 194.
19. Fishbein, *Crusading Obstetrician*, 211.
20. Ibid., 212.
21. Quoted in Fishbein, *Crusading Obstetrician*, 216–217.
22. Arnold R. Hirsch, *Making the Second Ghetto:Race and Housing in Chicago,1940-1960* (Cambridge: Cambridge University Press, 1983), 24; Beatrix Hoffman, *Health Care for Some: Rights and Rationing in the United States since 1930* (Chicago: University of Chicago Press 2012), 8.
23. Hirsch, *Making the Second Ghetto*, 24; Hoffman, *Health Care for Some*, 8.
24. Hoffman, *Health Care for Some*, 9.
25. Quoted in *The Chicago Maternity Center Story* https://www.kartemquin.com/films/the-chicago-maternity-center-story.
26. Quoted in Fishbein, *Crusading Obstetrician*, 212–13.
27. Chicago Maternity Center, First Annual Report (Chicago, 1933).
28. "Recollections: An Interview with Dr. Beatrice Tucker," by Diane Redleaf and Pat Kelleher, in *Health & Medicine*, vol. 1, issue 4 (1983), Chicago Maternity Center Collection, Northwestern Memorial Hospital Archives, Chicago, Illinois. This collection does not have a complete finding guide or catalog, and boxes are not numbered.
29. Chicago Maternity Center, First Annual Report (Chicago, 1933), 27.
30. Ibid.
31. DeLee, "Report of the Chairman," in Chicago Maternity Center, *Fourth Annual Report* (Chicago, 1936), 5.
32. Lynn Weiner, "Reconstructing Motherhood: The La Leche League in Postwar America," *The Journal of American History* (1994) 80(4): 1366.
33. DeLee, "Report of the Chairman," in Chicago Maternity Center, *Ninth Annual Report* (Chicago, 1941), 8.
34. DeLee's own biographer was not able to offer an explanation for it, acknowledging that DeLee's claims of the benefits of home births were "obviously . . . an argument against maternity hospitals, but who expects a crusader to be completely logical?" Fishbein, 212.
35. In her influential work *Brought to Bed*, Judith Walzer Leavitt discusses DeLee's concerns about puerperal fever epidemics in maternity wards, and his demands to restructure hospitals in order to protect laboring women from the dangers of infection: Leavitt, *Brought to Bed* (1988; repr. New York: Oxford University Press, 2016), 186.
36. See Jacqueline H. Wolf, *Deliver Me from Pain: Anesthesia and Birth in America* (Baltimore: Johns Hopkins University Press, 2009), 82.
37. As historian Charlotte Borst argues, "the standards of scientific, male professionalism were presumed to be absolutely essential for white women, but a black female midwife, properly supervised by the state, was considered adequate for black women." *Catching Babies*, 157.
38. Chicago Maternity Center, Annual Report (Chicago, 1949).
39. Chicago Maternity Center, Ninth Annual Report (Chicago, 1951).

40. Interview by Jacqueline H. Wolf of retired obstetrician, July 19, 2004, Winnetka.

41. Chicago Maternity Center, Annual Report (Chicago, 1952).

42. Brooks Ranney, "Responsibilities, Ten Problems, and a Few Solutions," *Obstetrics and Gynecology* 61, no. 2 (1983): 245.

43. Carol Leonard, *Lady's Hands, Lion's Heart: A Midwife's Saga* (Hopkinton: Bad Beaver Publishing, 2010), p. 25.

44. M. Edward Davis and Mabel C. Carmon, *DeLee's Obstetrics for Nurses*, 13th edition (Philadelphia: W. B. Saunders, 1944), 180.

45. Ibid., 181.

46. Ibid.

47. Ibid., 185.

48. Joseph B. DeLee, *Obstetrics for Nurses*, 9th ed. (Philadelphia: W. B. Saunders, 1930), 162; Patricia D'Antonio, *American Nursing: A History of Knowledge, Authority, and the Meaning of Work* (Baltimore: Johns Hopkins University Press, 2010), 41.

49. Chicago Maternity Center, Annual Report (Chicago, 1954).

50. For more on the negative experiences of women attempting natural childbirth in a hospital setting, see Wolf, *Deliver Me from Pain*, chapter 3.

51. Weiner, "Reconstructing Motherhood," 1365.

52. In *Back to the Breast: Natural Motherhood and Breastfeeding in America* (University of Chicago Press, 2015), Jessica Martucci argues that despite being in the minority, breastfeeding advocates at mid-century successfully "cultivated, manipulated, and spread knowledge about breastfeeding among themselves," ultimately creating "legitimacy and validation for their perspective" by drawing on a small group of doctors and scientists researching the benefits of breastfeeding (p. 2).

53. Martucci points out that most historical treatments of La Leche League portray the organization as either a conservative attempt "to reinstate a Victorian vision of motherhood" or a "false start" to the feminist movement of the 1960s and 1970s (*Back to the Breast*, 11). Martucci and Weiner both offer nuanced portrayals of the organization.

54. Weiner, "Reconstructing Motherhood," 1375.

55. For an excellent history of breastfeeding in the United States focused on debates surrounding science and motherhood, see Martucci, *Back to the Breast*.

56. Weiner, "Reconstructing Motherhood," 1360.

57. Robert Mendelsohn, *Confessions of a Medical Heretic* (Chicago: Contemporary Books, 1979), 92.

58. Ibid., 107.

59. Marian Tompson and Melissa Clark Vickers, *Passionate Journey: My Unexpected Life* (Amarillo, TX: Praeclarus Press, 2016), 50.

60. Marian Tompson, "Custom-Made Delivery," in Dave and Lee Stewart, eds., *Safe Alternatives in Childbirth, Based on the First American NAPSAC Conference* (Marble Hill, MO: NAPSAC Reproductions, 1976), 207.

61. Grantly Dick-Read, *The Natural Childbirth Primer* (New York: Harper and Row, 1955), 1.

62. Marian Tompson interview with author, December 23, 2015, Chicago, IL.

63. Tompson and Vickers, *Passionate Journey*, 66.

64. Tompson and Vickers, *Passionate Journey*, 67.

65. Correspondence between Tompson and Dick-Read. Marian's letter has no date, but Dick-Read's response is dated Oct 23, 1957. Box 87, correspondence and memos 1957–69, La Leche League International Records (LLLI), DePaul University Archives, Chicago, IL.

66. Weiner, "Reconstructing Motherhood," 1362.

67. Ibid., 1357.

68. Paula Michaels, *Lamaze: An International History* (New York: Oxford University Press, 2014), 21.

69. Ibid.

70. Barbara Katz Rothman, *In Labor: Women and Power in the Birthplace* (New York: Norton, 1991), 79.

71. Barbara Katz Rothman, "Laboring Then," in *Laboring On: Birth in Transition in the United States* (New York: Routledge 2007), 23.

72. Marian Tompson, "Custom-Made Delivery," 207.

73. Author interview with Marian Tompson, December 23, 2015.

74. Tompson, "Custom-Made Delivery," 207.

75. Helen Ratner Dietz, "Herbert Ratner, MD and Gregory White, MD: Pioneer Advocates of Maternal-Child Health," paper presented at the Integritas Institute Bio-Ethics Seminar Lecture Series, University of Illinois Chicago (February 11, 2015), 7.

76. Gregory White and Mayer Eisenstein, "The American College of Home Obstetrics (ACHO): Philosophy and Practice of Physicians in Homebirth," in David Stewart and Lee Stewart, eds., *21st Century Obsterics Now!* Vol. 2 (NAPSAC 1977), 360.

77. Ibid.

78. Helen Ratner Dietz, "Herbert Ratner, MD and Gregory White, MD," 8.

79. Author interview with Kay Furey, June 2, 2015.

80. White and Eisenstein, "The American College of Home Obstetrics," 361.

81. Interestingly, Joseph DeLee noted that he charged more for a home delivery than a C-section because of the extra time involved.

82. Mayer Eisenstein, *The Home Birth Advantage* (Chicago: CMI Press, 2000), p. 9

83. White comments, 1964 LLLI convention, panel on childbirth, p. 9. LLLI Records.

84. Ibid., 10.

85. Quoted in Weiner, "Reconstructing Motherhood," 1368.

86. "Viewpoint: Herbert Ratner, MD," reprinted from THE D.O., July 1967, volume 7 no. 11, no page numbers, 11.37, LLLI Records.

87. Tompson keynote address September 20, 1975, Iowa area meeting, 87.5, LLLI Records.

88. Ibid.

89. La Leche League International, *The Womanly Art of Breastfeeding*, 2nd edition (London: Tandem, 1971), 53.

90. Transcript, proceedings, second biennial convention, June 22–24, 1966, Indianapolis, IN, LLLI Records.

91. Weiner, "Reconstructing Motherhood," 1359.

92. In 1964 the total number was 2,132; 1965 it was 1,844, and in 1966, the number was down to 1,700.

93. In 1960, the census reported 788 "White" residents in the Near West Side neighborhood, 68,146 "Negro," and 57,676 "other races." According to the *Electronic Encyclopedia of Chicago*, "African Americans and Mexicans moved into the Near West Side in larger numbers during the 1930s and 1940s. Approximately 26,000 African Americans lived there by 1940, with the number increasing to more than 68,000 by 1960, in part due to the "Great Migration" of black southerners. On the West Side as a whole the African American community grew rapidly during the 1940s and 1950s, as residential opportunities remained largely limited to ghettoes on the South and West Sides," See http://www.encyclopedia.chicagohistory.org/pages/878.html.

94. Hirsch, *Making the Second Ghetto*, 24.

95. Tucker to Dr. Richard Kessler, March 3, 1971, Beatrice Tucker Correspondence, CMC papers.

96. "Recollections: An Interview with Dr. Beatrice Tucker," Beatrice Tucker Correspondence, CMC papers.

97. Patricia Krizmis and Angela Parker, "Roaches Watch Birth in a Slum Apartment," *Chicago Tribune*, June 21, 1971. CMC papers.

98. Tim Hunter, "Ward Rounds," http://www.wardrounds.northwestern.edu/2012/10/training-at-the-chicago-maternity-center/.

99. David Kerns, *Fortnight on Maxwell Street* (Point Richmond: Bay Tree Publishing, 2018), 42, 80. *Fortnight on Maxwell Street* is a historical novel based on Kerns' experiences as a resident at the CMC in 1968.

100. http://www.wardrounds.northwestern.edu/2012/10/training-at-the-chicago-maternity-center/.

101. Ibid.

102. Hirsch, *Making the Second Ghetto*, 269.

103. Quoted in Hoffman, *Health Care for Some,* 144.

104. Chicago Maternity Center, *Annual Report* (Chicago, 1966/67), transcript of radio program, "The Talk of Chicago," with commentator Mal Bellairs.

105. Hirsch, *Making the Second Ghetto*, 269.

106. RAM position paper, January 1968, quoted in Robert Geoelli, *Environmental Activism and the Urban Crisis: Baltimore, St. Louis, Chicago* (Philadelphia: Temple University Press, 2014), 83.

107. See Natalie Y. Moore, *The South Side: A Portrait of Chicago and American Segregation* (New York: St. Martin's Press, 2016), 87.

108. http://www.uic.edu/depts/uichistory/.

109. Chicago Maternity Center, *Annual Report* (Chicago, 1966/67).

110. David Danforth, "Women's Hospital and Maternity Center Scheduled to Open in 1972," brochure, ND, c. 1970, Beatrice Tucker, M.D., Correspondence, c. 1940–1972, Chicago Maternity Center Collection.

111. Tucker to Bayly, June 22, 1972, Beatrice Tucker, M.D., Correspondence, c. 1940–1972.

112. Tucker to Danforth, ND, Beatrice Tucker, M.D., Correspondence, c. 1940–1972.

113. http://www.dezeen.com/2014/10/02/prentice-womens-hospital-chicago-by-bertrand-goldberg-associates-brutalism/.

114. Telephone conversation with Rhona Jacobs, January 26, 2016.

115. Mayer Eisenstein, *The Home Birth Advantage*, 13.

116. Author interview with Kay Furey, June 2, 2015.

117. Obstetric Records, Furey personal collection.

118. Furey was initially interested in going to medical school but she did not get in. She obtained a BSN from Loyola and a Masters of Science at University of Illinois Chicago so that she could open an independent practice.

119. Author interview with Paul Schattauer, December 23, 2015.

120. "Homefirst News," Special Edition (1989), 2: Furey personal collection.

121. "Homefirst News," Special Edition (1989), 2.

122. "Homefirst News," Special Edition (1989), 4.

123. "WBEZ Radio Interview—9/1986," in "Alternative Childbirth Film and Discussion Seminars," Homefirst Family Health Services (Winter/Spring schedule, 1987), Furey personal collection.

124. "Homefirst Health Services" flier, ND, Furey personal collection.

125. "Homefirst News," vol 2 no. 1 (1988), 6, Furey personal collection.

126. Author interview with Kay Furey, June 2015.

127. Eisenstein, *The Home Birth Advantage*, 130–131.

128. Ibid., 193–196.

129. "Homefirst News," vol 2 no. 1 (1988), 5.

130. Author interview with Schattauer, December 23, 2015.

CHAPTER 2

1. Judith Rooks, *Midwifery and Childbirth in America* (Philadelphia: Temple University Press, 1997), 60.

2. Lawrence Feinberg, "Some Find Birth at Home 'Beautiful,'" *The Washington Post*, April 13, 1975, p. B1.

3. Helen Morarre quoted in Lawrence Feinberg, "Some Find Birth at Home 'Beautiful,'" *The Washington Post*, April 13, 1975, p. B1.

4. Fran Ventre quoted in Lawrence Feinberg, "Some Find Birth at Home 'Beautiful,'" *The Washington Post*, April 13, 1975, p. B2.

5. Marion McCartney, interview with author, December 13, 2011.

6. For more on the changing role of fathers in childbirth, see Judith Walzer Leavitt, *Make Room for Daddy: The Journey from Waiting Room to Birthing Room* (Chapel Hill: University of North Carolina Press, 2010).

7. https://www.washingtonpost.com/archive/local/1999/10/25/obituaries/146425f5-7b94-4109-bf84-cc7f34a13111/.

8. Quoted in Stephan Schwartz, "A Holy War Rages over Natural Childbirth," *Washington Post Potomac*, 48.

9. Quoted in Schwartz, "A Holy War," 39.

10. Ibid.

11. My sister was delivered by Dr. Sachs, in 1964, while my mother was unconscious. Sachs reported that by 1978 at least 75 percent of women were awake for their births at Holy Cross. See Penelope Lemov, "Childbirth: A Weekly Guide to Current Approaches to Childbirth and Study Courses Available to Expectant Parents," *Washington Post Maryland Weekly*, January 5, 1978, 1.

12. Marion McCartney, interview with author December 13, 2011.

13. Quoted in Schwartz, "A Holy War," 12.

14. Ibid., 51.

15. Robert F. Levey, "Natural Birth: The Agony and Ecstasy," *The Washington Post*, May 28, 1972, D1–D2.

16. Ibid.

17. Jane Murphy, "Teacher Training," ASPO news Washington, D.C. area chapter, June 1975, p. 2; Esther Herman personal collection.

18. Alice Bailes, letter "To All in D.C. ASPO," *Special Delivery*, November 1, 1972, Esther Herman personal collection.

19. Marsha Jackson, "You Need Two Clamps and a Pair of Scissors," in Geradine Simkins, ed. *Into These Hands: Wisdom from Midwives* (Traverse City, MI: Spirituality and Health Books, 2011), 128.

20. "Doctors are finding themselves upstaged," *Washington Post Potomac*, October 18, 1970, 50.

21. Fran Ventre, "Special Delivery: Newsletter of the Professional and Physicians Divisions," Washington, D.C. ASPO November 1972, 1–2. Herman personal collection.

22. *News from H.O.M.E.* 2, no. 2 (Spring 1977): 2, Fran Ventre Papers, 1970–2000; MC 772, Folder 8.2. Schlesinger Library, Radcliffe Institute, Harvard University, Cambridge, MA.

23. Fran Ventre and Esther Herman, interview with author, October 28, 2011.

24. Up until that point, according to Phyllis Stein, all ASPO teachers had to have an MD or an RN.

25. Phyllis Stein, interview with author, July 15, 2016 (via Skype).

26. See Paula Michaels, "The Sights and Sounds of Natural Childbirth: Films and Records in Antenatal Preparation Classes, 1950s–1980s," *Social History of Medicine* 31 no. 1 (February 2018), 24–40.

27. Fran Ventre and Esther Herman, interview with author, October 28, 2011.

28. "Blizzard Snarls East," *Milwaukee Sentinel*, January 31, 1966, p. 1. https://news.google.com/newspapers?nid=wZJMF1LD7PcC&dat=19660131&printsec=frontpage&hl=en.

29. Fran Ventre, email correspondence with author, July 13, 2016.

30. Fran Ventre and Esther Herman, interview with author, October 28, 2011.

31. Diana Kohn quoted in https://www.washingtonpost.com/local/md-politics/a-post-hippie-takoma-park/2012/07/07/gJQAXgtSUW_story.html.

32. Fran Ventre and Esther Herman, interview with author, October 28, 2011.

33. Herman quoted in Susan Seliger, "Home is Where More Births Are," *The National Observer*, January 15, 1977, p. 14.

34. Fran Ventre and Esther Herman, interview with author, October 28, 2011.

35. Herman quoted in Selinger, "Home is Where More Births Are," p. 14.

36. Fran Ventre and Esther Herman, interview with author, July 25, 2011.

37. Blue Ridge Potomac LLL Manual 1975, Box 89, "MD/DE/DC Leaders Guidebook 1975" folder, La Leche League International Records (LLLI) DePaul University Archives, Chicago, IL.

38. Ibid., 1.

39. Esther Herman, email correspondence with author, July 13, 2016.

40. Fran Ventre and Esther Herman, interview with author, October 28, 2011.

41. Esther Herman, email correspondence with author, July 13, 2016.

42. Fran Ventre, "The Making of a Legalized Lay Midwife," *News from Home* 1, no. 2 (April 1976): 3, Folder 8.2, Fran Ventre Papers

43. Fran Ventre, interview with author, June 14, 2016.

44. Ibid.

45. For more on the consumer health movement of the 1970s, see Nancy Tomes, *Remaking the American Patient: How Madison Avenue and Modern Medicine Turned Patients into Consumers* (Chapel Hill: University of North Carolina Press, 2016).

46. Fran Ventre, interview with author, June 14, 2016.

47. Alice Bailes, interview with author, December 14, 2011.

48. Alice Bailes, "The Knowledge in Your Hands," in *Into These Hands*, pp. 28–29.

49. Jan Epstein, quoted in Anne Kasper, "Independent Practice as a Nurse Midwife in Bethesda, Maryland: An Interview with Jan Epstein, CNM," *Women and Health*, Vol. 6(3/4), Fall/Winter 1981, p. 177.

50. Esther Herman, letter to the Editor, *Washington Star-News*, December 21, 1974, p. A-11.

51. Fran Ventre and Esther Herman, interview with author, October 28, 2011.

52. Sheilah Kast, "Rare is the Area Doctor Who Does Home Deliveries," *Washington Star-News*, December 2, 1974, p. B2.

53. Esther Herman, letter to the Editor, *Washington Star-News*, December 21, 1974, p. A-11.

54. Marlene Miller, "Controversial Home Deliveries Rising," *The Alexandria Gazette*, October 11, 1974, p. 5-A.

55. Lawrence Feinberg, "Some Find Birth at Home 'Beautiful,'" *The Washington Post*, April 13, 1975, p. B1–2. Herman personal collection.

56. Joy Billington, "Births at Home," *Washington Star Portfolio*, Jan 4, 1976, pp. D1–D2.

57. James Brew, quoted in Joy Billington, "Births at Home," *Washington Star Portfolio*, p. D1–D2.

58. Fran Ventre and Esther Herman, interview with author, October 28, 2011.

59. Fran Ventre, interview with author June 14, 2016. Schwab's story ended tragically, however; in 1976, suffering from depression, he committed suicide by jumping off of the Woodrow Wilson Bridge.

60. Dorothea M. Lang, "The Midwife Returns—Modern Style," reprinted from *Parents' Magazine*, October 1972, 1, Herman personal collection.

61. Ibid.

62. This is part of trend, beginning in the mid-1960s, to have advanced practice nurses (and physician assistants) take on new clinical roles left unfilled by shortages of physicians. See Julie Fairman, *Making Room in the Clinic: Nurse Practitioners and the Evolution of Modern Health Care* (New Brunswick: Rutgers University Press, 2009).

63. Rooks, *Midwifery and Childbirth in America*, 69.

64. See Winifred Connerton and Patricia D'Antonio, "International Comparisons: The Nursing-Midwifery Interface," in Anne Borsay and Billie Hunter, eds., *Nursing and Midwifery in Britain since 1700* (Basingstoke: Palgrave 2012), p. 189.

65. Rooks, *Midwifery and Childbirth in America*, 70–71.

66. Connerton and D'Antonio, "International Comparisons," p. 190. For a complete history of nurse-midwifery, see Laura E. Ettinger, *Nurse-Midwifery: The Birth of a New American Profession* (Columbus: Ohio State University Press, 2006); Helen Varney and Joyce Beebe Thompson, *The Midwife Said Fear Not: A History of Midwifery in the United States* (New York: Springer, 2016). See also Judy Barrett Litoff, *The American Midwife Debate: A Sourcebook on its Modern Origins* (Toronto: Praeger, 1986).

67. Alice Bailes, interview with author, December 14, 2011.

68. Alice Bailes, "The Knowledge in Your Hands," in *Into These Hands*, p. 28.

69. Joy Billington, "Births at Home," *Washington Star Portfolio*, p. D1–D2.

70. James Brew, quoted in Joy Billington, "Births at Home," *Washington Star Portfolio*, p. D1–D2

71. Ibid.

72. Jan Epstein, quoted in Anne Kasper, "Independent Practice as a Nurse Midwife in Bethesda, Maryland," p. 178.

73. Fran Ventre, "The Making of a Legalized Lay Midwife," p. 4.

74. Phyllis Stein, interview with author, July 15, 2016 (via Skype).

75. Alice Bailes, "The Knowledge in Your Hands," in *Into These Hands*, p. 28.

76. Gene Declercq, interview with author, October 11, 2016.

77. Fran Ventre, "The Making of a Legalized Lay Midwife," p. 5.

78. Ibid.

79. Katy Dawley, "Leaving the Nest: Nurse-Midwifery in the United States, 1940–1980" (PhD dissertation, University of Pennsylvania, 2001), p. 322.

80. Fran Ventre, "The Making of a Legalized Lay Midwife," p. 6.

81. Ibid., p. 7.

82. Ventre, "The Making of a Legalized Lay Midwife," p. 7.

83. In 1981, there were 4200 Fellows in District IV, representing approximately 18 percent of College membership. Reported at Annual District Meeting, Walt Disney World, 1982, A.C.O.G. Records, 6/G/4/District IV/2000/7.4, American College of Obstetricians and Gynecologists Library, Washington, D.C.

84. ACOG District IV Minutes, Interim Advisory Council Meeting, March 8–9, 1980, Atlanta, GA, p. 11.

85. Guy Meares, Advisory Council Meeting—District IV, A.C.O.G. Headquarters, Washington, D.C., March 5–6, 1983, p. 17.

86. Vernon R. Randall to Fran Ventre, January 27, 1976, Folder 7.2.

87. ACOG district IV minutes, Interim Advisory Council Meeting, Atlanta, GA, March 8-9, 1980, p. 23.

88. Fran Ventre, testimony against HB 228, MC 772, Folder 12.7. Emphasis in original.

89. Ibid.

90. Until the bill passed, Maryland was one of only six states that forbade non-nurse midwives to attend home births. https://rewire.news/article/2015/05/12/maryland-legalizes-homebirths-midwives/.

91. Ibid.

92. Fran Ventre, testimony against HB 228, p. 4.

93. Patricia D'Antonio, *American Nursing: A History of Knowledge, Authority, and the Meaning of Work* (Baltimore: Johns Hopkins Press, 2010), pp. 169–170.

94. Fran Ventre and Esther Herman, interview with author, October 28, 2011. The introduction of the associate degree programs in nursing was part of the shift of nursing education into universities and colleges after WWII, as a way to increase the production of nurses. While the ADN programs prepared RNs, if nurses wanted to practice as clinical nurse specialists/advance practice nurses, they would need to get the BSN and then post-baccalaureate or a Masters. See Patricia D'Antonio, *American Nursing*, ch. 7.

95. Fran Ventre and Esther Herman, interview with author, October 28, 2011.

96. See Martin Summers, *Madness in the City of Magnificent Intentions: A History of Race and Mental Illness in the Nation's Capital* (forthcoming).

97. Gregory J. Ahart Testimony before the House Committee on District of Columbia: Fiscal and Governmental Affairs Committee, March 28, 1977, p. 4. http://www.gao.gov/assets/100/98417.pdf.

98. Ibid., p. 1.

99. Ibid., p. 13.

100. Fran Ventre, "Reaction Log," January 29, 1976, MC 772 Folder 3.4.

101. Ibid.

102. Ventre, "Reaction Log," February 19, 1976.

103. Ventre, Reaction Log, January 29, 1976.

104. Summers, *Madness in the City of Magnificent Intentions,* (forthcoming), p. 2.

105. Ibid., ch. 10 p. 3.

106. Ventre, "Reaction Log," March 11, 1976.

107. Ventre, "Reaction Log," March 4, 1976.

108. Ventre, "Reaction Log," February 5, 1976.

109. Ann Lohn and Jo Weisbrod, "Dance/Movement Therapy Program at St. Elizabeths Hospital," MC 772, Folder 3.4, 1.

110. Ventre, "Reaction Log," February 19, 1976.

111. Ibid.

112. Ibid.

113. Ventre, "Reaction Log," March 4, 1976.

114. Ventre, "Reaction Log," March 11, 1976.

115. Ventre, "Parent Education Course Design," MC 772, Folder 3.4, p. 4.

116. Fran Ventre and Esther Herman, interview with author, October 28, 2011.

117. Attempts at clarifying midwifery legislation began in earnest in 1977 with a proposed clarification/ amendment coming from the District of Columbia Register. See "Proposed Rulemaking: Commission on Licensure to Practice the Health Art," ACNM Records (43.18).

118. Ibid.

119. "Report of Self-Evaluation Prepared by the Faculty of the Nurse Midwifery Program of the School of Nursing of Georgetown University" submitted to the ACNM, March 1975, p. 61, ACNM records, MSC 330a (7.26), National Library of Medicine, Bethesda, MD.

120. Ibid.

121. Marion McCartney, interview with author December 13, 2011.

122. Ibid.

123. Ibid.

124. Ibid.

125. "Report of Self-Evaluation Prepared by the Faculty of the Nurse Midwifery Program of the School of Nursing of Georgetown University," March 1975, p. 58.

126. Shargel quoted in Jacob Fenston, "From Public Hospital to Homeless Shelter: the Long History of DC General." May 30, 2014. WAMU broadcast. http://wamu.org/programs/metro_connection/14/05/30/from_public_hospital_to_homeless_shelter_the_long_history_of_dc_general.

127. "Report of Self-Evaluation Prepared by the Faculty of the Nurse Midwifery Program of the School of Nursing of Georgetown University" submitted to the ACNM, March 1975, ACNM records 33a 7.26.

128. Eileen Sheil, "Final Report, DC General Hospital Nurse Midwifery Service, 10/29/73–10/31/74," ACNM Records (43.18).

129. Ibid.

130. Marion McCartney and Jan Epstein, interview with author, October 26, 2011.

131. Persis, letter to Fran Ventre, February 23, 1996; Ventre papers, Folder 6.9.

132. Michele Nylund, letter to Fran Ventre, ND, Ventre papers, Folder 6.9.

133. Ellen, Steve, and Alicia Anzian, letter to Fran Ventre, April 1, 1996; Ventre papers, Folder 6.9.

134. Jan Epstein, quoted in Anne Kasper, *Women and Health*, p. 180.

135. Marsha Jackson, "You Need Two Clamps and a Pair of Scissors," p. 128.

136. Marion McCartney and Jan Epstein, interview with author, October 26, 2011.

137. Joy Billington, "Births at Home," *Washington Star*, January 4, 1976, p. D1.

138. Marion McCartney and Jan Epstein, interview with author, October 26, 2011.

139. Quoted in Joy Billington, "Births at Home," *Washington Star*, January 4, 1976, p. D2.

140. Ibid.

141. Ibid.

142. Marion McCartney, interview with author December 13, 2011.

143. Durrin Films, Inc., flier, ACNM Records, MSC 330A, 11.41.

144. Dawley, "Leaving the Nest: Nurse-Midwifery in the United States, 1940–1980," pp. 322–323.

145. "Daughters of Time," ACNM Records.

146. Ventre and Herman, interview with author, July 25, 2011.

147. Herman, Miller-Klein, and Ventre, "A Survey of Current Trends in Home Birth," in Stewart and Stewart, eds., *Compulsory Hospitalization: Freedom of Choice in Childbirth?* Vol. 3 (Marble Hill: NAPSAC Reproductions, 1979), p. 759.

148. Connerton and D'Antonio, "International Comparisons: The Nursing-Midwifery Interface," p. 190.

CHAPTER 3

1. Joanne Santana, lecture, The Farm Midwifery Assistant Workshop, Summertown, TN, March 26, 2013.

2. Ibid.

3. Stephen Gaskin, *The Caravan*, rev. ed. (1972; Summertown, TN: Book Publishing Co., 2007), 127.

4. Stephen Gaskin, *Monday Night Class*, rev. ed. (Summertown, TN: Book Publishing Co., 2005), 8.

5. There is a vast and expanding literature on the history of psychedelic psychiatry. See in particular Erika Dyck, *Psychedelic Psychiatry: LSD from Clinic to Campus* (Baltimore: Johns Hopkins University Press, 2008); Matthew Oram, "The Trials of Psychedelic Medicine: LSD Psychotherapy, Clinical Science, and Pharmaceutical Regulation in the United States," PhD diss., University of Sydney, 2014.

6. Melvyn Stiriss, *Voluntary Peasants: Labor of Love* (Warwick, NY: Hot Button Press, 2012) location 679 (Kindle).

7. Joanne Santana, lecture, The Farm Midwifery Assistant Workshop, Summertown, TN, March 26, 2013.
8. David Talbot, *Season of the Witch: Enchantment, Terror, and Deliverance in the City of Love* (New York: Simon and Schuster, 2012), 158.
9. Timothy Miller, *The Hippies and American Values* (Knoxville: University of Tennessee Press, 1991), 16.
10. Warren James Belasco, *Appetite for Change: How the Counterculture Took on the Food Industry* (Ithaca: Cornell University Press, 2006), 97.
11. Santana lecture, The Farm Midwifery Assistant Workshop, Summertown, TN, March 26, 2013.
12. Leo Eloesser, "Assembly Line for Country Midwives," *Pacific Spectator* 7, no. 2 (Spring 1953): 2.
13. J.E.B. McPhail, "Summary of CLARA-UNICEF Medical Program in North China," February 6, 1950, MSS 20 Folder 2, Box 20, Leo Eloesser Papers, Lane Medical Archives, Stanford University Medical Center (hereafter cited as Eloesser Papers).
14. Eloesser, "Assembly Line for Country Midwives," 2.
15. Ibid., 2–7.
16. Press Release ICEF/201, April 5, 1950, United Nations Department of Public Information Press and Publications Bureau, Box 20 Folder 2, Eloesser Papers.
17. According to Victor and Ruth Sidel, by 1972 there were over 1,000,000 barefoot doctors in China. See Victor Sidel and Ruth Sidel, *Serve the People: Observations on Medicine in the People's Republic of China* (Beacon Press, 1973), 197. An American translation of *A Barefoot Doctor's Manual* was first published in the United States in 1974 by the U.S. Department of Health, Education, and Welfare (Public Health Service, National Institutes of Health, Bethesda, MD, in series: DHEW publication no. (NIH) 75–695; translation of Ch'ih chiao i sheng shou ts'e) and appealed to many American readers interested in a basic reference guide to Chinese medicine, including descriptions of acupuncture, massage, and herbal treatments. Four pages cover "New Methods for Delivery of the Newborn"— nothing in comparison to what readers could find in Eloesser's *Pregnancy, Childbirth and the Newborn* or in Ina May Gaskin's *Spiritual Midwifery*.
18. Amanda Harris, S. Belton, L. Barclay, and J Fenwick, "Midwives in China: 'jie sheng po' to 'zhu chan shi,'" *Midwifery* 25 (2009): 205.
19. Harris et. al., "Midwives in China," 203–212.
20. Eloesser, "Assembly Line for Country Midwives," 3.
21. J.E.B. McPhail, "Summary of CLARA-UNICEF Medical Program in North China," 2.
22. Isabel Hemingway to Leo Eloesser, April 24, 1955, Folder 2, Box 15, Eloesser papers.
23. Nicholas Eastman to Leo Eloesser, October 5, 1956 Folder 2, Box 15, Eloesser papers.
24. Victor Richards to Leo Eloesser, January 30, 1973, Folder 2, Box 15, Eloesser papers.
25. September 1975 interview with Carol Downer and Santa Cruz Midwives, Downer personal collection.
26. Melvyn Stiriss, *Voluntary Peasants: Labor of Love*, location 1342.
27. Santana, lecture, The Farm Midwifery Assistant Workshop, Summertown, TN, March 26, 2013.
28. Ibid.
29. Ina May Gaskin, "Birth Story: A 'Pregnancy' 30 Years in the Making," http://www.huffingtonpost.com/ina-may-gaskin/post_4689_b_3253016.html, May 10, 2013.
30. Ina May Gaskin quoted in Katie Allison Granju, "The Midwife of Modern Midwifery," June 1, 1999, http://www.salon.com/1999/06/01/gaskin/.
31. Ina May Gaskin, conversation with author, March 26, 2013.
32. Ibid.
33. Gwyn Harvey, "Interview with Pamela Hunt," *Birth Gazette* Vol. 4 No. 1 (Fall 1987), p. 6.

34. "Pamela's Story," in Gaskin, *Spiritual Midwifery*, 4th ed. (Summertown, TN: Book Publishing Co., 2002), 22.
35. Harvey, "Interview with Pamela Hunt," 6.
36. Pamela Hunt, interview with the author, March 29, 2013.
37. Cara Gillette, email correspondence with author, August 24, 2013.
38. Gaskin, *The Caravan*, 14.
39. Ibid., 35.
40. Ibid., 165.
41. "Street" drugs such as speed and heroin were strictly forbidden on the Caravan.
42. Gaskin, *The Caravan*, 83.
43. Ibid., 22.
44. Michael Traugot, quoted in Gaskin, *The Caravan*, 170.
45. Ibid., 171.
46. Cara Gillette, email correspondence with the author, August 24, 2013.
47. Gaskin, *Spiritual Midwifery* (2002), 17.
48. "Pamela's Story," in Gaskin, *Spiritual Midwifery* (2002), 23.
49. Gaskin, *Spiritual Midwifery* (2002), 16.
50. Cara Gillette, email correspondence with the author, August 24, 2013.
51. "Anne's Birth," in Gaskin, *Spiritual Midwifery* (2002), 36.
52. Cara Gillette, email correspondence with the author, August 24, 2013.
53. "Pamela's Story," in Gaskin, *Spiritual Midwifery* (2002), 24.
54. Mary Fjerstad, email correspondence with the author, August 21, 2013.
55. "Anne's Birth," in Gaskin, *Spiritual Midwifery*, 36.
56. "Pamela's Story," in Gaskin, *Spiritual Midwifery* (2002), 24.
57. "Anne's Birth," in Gaskin, *Spiritual Midwifery*, 37.
58. Cara Gillette, email correspondence with the author, August 24, 2013.
59. "Pamela's Story," in Gaskin, *Spiritual Midwifery* (2002), 24.
60. Cara Gillette, email correspondence with the author, August 24, 2013.
61. "Pamela's Story," in Gaskin, *Spiritual Midwifery* (2002), 24.
62. Cara Gillette, email correspondence with the author, August 24, 2013.
63. Ina May Gaskin, *Spiritual Midwifery* (2002), 17.
64. Nancy Burns-Fusaro, "Dante Society Honors Four 'Bologna Boys,'" *Westerly Sun*, November 22, 2008.
65. Margaret Nofziger decided she did not want to continue studying or practicing midwifery after the Caravan.
66. Ina May Gaskin, conversation with author, March, 26, 2013.
67. "Farm Report January 1975," Phil Schweitzer private collection, Summertown, TN.
68. Ina May Gaskin, "Spiritual Midwifery," in *Hey Beatnik!* (Summertown, TN: Book Publishing Company, 1974), no pagination. Hazrat Inayat Kahn is the Sufi founder.
69. Rupert Fike, Cynthia Holzapfel, Albert Bates, Michael Cook, *Voices from The Farm: Adventures in Community Living*, 2nd ed. (Summertown, TN: Book Publishing Company, 2012), 12.
70. Fred Turner, *From Counterculture to Cyberculture: Stewart Brand, the Whole Earth Network, and the Rise of Digital Utopianism* (Chicago: University of Chicago Press, 2006), 32–33.
71. Albert K. Bates, "Technological Innovation in a Rural Intentional Community, 1971–1987," presented at the National Historic Communal Societies Association Annual Meeting, October 17, 1987, Bishop Hill, IL.
72. Phil Schweitzer, interview with the author, March 30, 2013.
73. Gaskin, *Spiritual Midwifery* (2002), 30.
74. Hunt, interview with the author, March 29, 2013.
75. Gaskin, *Spiritual Midwifery* (2002), 20.

76. Pamela Hunt, lecture, The Farm Midwifery Assistant Workshop, March 26, 2013, Summertown, TN.
77. (2002), 29.
78. "Pamela's Story," in Gaskin, *Spiritual Midwifery,*(2002), 26–27.
79. http://www.tributes.com/show/John-O.-Williams-88512246.
80. Posted by: Debbie O'Neal, August 21, 2003, http://www.tributes.com/condolences/view_memories/88512246?p=10&start_index=1.
81. John Williams to Ina May Gaskin, August 24, 1993. Letter in Pamela's Hunt's possession.
82. Ina May Gaskin, "Spiritual Midwifery," selection from *Hey Beatnik!* (N.P.)
83. Santana, lecture, The Farm Midwifery Assistant Workshop, March 26, 2013.
84. http://www.thefarmmidwives.org/preliminary_statistics.html (accessed May 30, 2013).
85. Hunt, interview with the author, March 29, 2013.
86. Ina May Gaskin conversation with author, March 26, 2013.
87. Although Ina May Gaskin is listed as the sole author of the book, many other midwives contributed to it as well.
88. This edition (original) doesn't have page numbers.
89. Gaskin, *Spiritual Midwifery* (1980), 70.
90. Ibid., 141.
91. Ibid., 63.
92. Lynda Bateman, Catriona Jones, and Julie Jomeen, "A Narrative Synthesis of Women's Out-of-Body Experiences During Childbirth," *Journal of Midwifery and Women's Health,* Vol. 62, No. 4, July/August 2017, p. 443.
93. Gaskin, *Spiritual Midwifery* (1980), 154.
94. Ibid., 62.
95. Walter Truett Anderson, *The Upstart Spring: Esalen and the Human Potential Movement: The First Twenty Years* (iuniverse, 2004), 66.
96. Abraham Maslow, *Religions, Values, and Peak Experiences* (Columbus: Ohio State University Press: 1964), 245. For more on Maslow, see Nadine Weidman, "Between the Counterculture and the Corporation: Abraham Maslow and Humanistic Psychology in the 1960s," in David Kaiser and W. Patrick McCray, eds., *Groovy Science: Knowledge, Innovation and American Counterculture* (Chicago: The University of Chicago Press, 2016), 109–141.
97. Gaskin, *Spiritual Midwifery* (1980), 142.
98. Stanislav Grof, "Varieties of Transpersonal Experiences: Observations from LSD Psychotherapy," *Journal of Transpersonal Psychology*, Vol. IV, No. 1, 1972, p. 51.
99. Gaskin, *Spiritual Midwifery* (1980), 153.
100. Ibid., 133.
101. Ibid., 77.
102. Grof, interview, "The Great Awakening," in Roger Walsh and Charles Grob, eds., *Higher Wisdom: Eminent Elders Explore the Continuing Impact of Psychedelics* (New York: SUNY Press, 2005), 122.
103. Grof, "Great Awakening," p. 123.
104. Grof interviewed in Keith Thompson, "Search for the Self," *Yoga Journal,* July/August 1990, p. 57.
105. Grof, "The Great Awakening," p. 120.
106. Jeffrey A. Lieberman, *Shrinks: The Untold Story of Psychiatry* (Boston: Back Bay Books, 2016), 106.
107. Grof, "Varieties of Transpersonal Experiences," *Journal of Transpersonal Psychology,* 1972, p. 47.
108. Martin Halliwell, *Therapeutic Revolutions: Medicine, Psychiatry, and American Culture, 1945–1970* (Rutgers University Press, 2014), p. 261.

109. Grof, "Implications of Psychedelic Research for Anthropology: Observations from LSD Psychotherapy" at conference "Ritual: Reconciliation in Change," July 21–29, 1973; Paper prepared in advance for participants in Burg Wartenstein Symposium No. 59, p. 8, Box 1, Folder 3, MSP 1, Stanislav Grof papers, Karnes Archives and Special Collections, Purdue University Libraries, West Lafayette, Indiana.
110. For more on the Maryland Psychiatric Research Institute studies, see Matthew Oram, "The Trials of Psychedelic Medicine," PhD diss., University of Sydney.
111. Subject 7, Box 1, Folder 7, MSP 170, Maryland Psychiatric Research Center LSD Professional Training Program Study files, Karnes Archives and Special Collections, Purdue University Libraries, West Lafayette, Indiana.
112. Subject 6, Box 1, MSP 170.
113. Subject 15, Box 1, MSP 170.
114. Subject 10, Box 1, MSP 170.
115. Subject 15, Box 1, MSP 170.
116. Grof, "The Great Awakening," p. 133.
117. Subject 18, Box 1, MSP 170.
118. In developing this theory, Grof was undoubtedly influenced by other psychiatrists who had focused on birth trauma, namely Otto Rank, and to some extent Sigmund Freud. Others began to focus on birth and primal therapy in the postwar era/1970s, such as Arthur Janov, but disagreed about what type of therapeutic effects would be successful.
119. Subject 18, Box 1, MSP 170.
120. Ibid.
121. Grof, "The Great Awakening," 133.
122. Grof, *The Adventure of Self-Discovery: Dimensions of Consciousness and New Perspectives in Psychotherapy and Inner Exploration* (New York: SUNY Press, 1988), p. 9.
123. Grof quoted in Jeffrey Kripal, *Esalen: America and the Religion of No Religion* (Chicago: University of Chicago Press, 2008), 258.
124. Midwives Raven Lang and Kate Bowland, featured in Chapter 4, frequently cited Grof's work. Bowland writes about him in her diary; Lang cites him in *Birth Book* (1972; repr., Felton, CA: Genesis Press, 2007), 39. Lang believes that Grof was the most influential of all social scientists whose work she studied (Lang email correspondence with author, January 25, 2015).

CHAPTER 4

1. Karen Ehrlich, interview with author, August 6, 2011.
2. Kristin Thomas, "First Day Discussions, Santa Cruz Midwives," September 1975, p. 86, Carol Downer personal collection.
3. Sheryl Burt Ruzek, *The Women's Health Movement: Feminist Alternatives to Medical Control* (Westport: Praeger, 1978), 59.
4. Much valuable scholarship exists on the issue of "choice" as a problematic concept with which to build bridges across race and class. See, for example, Dorothy Roberts, *Killing the Black Body: Race, Reproduction, and the Meaning of Liberty* (New York: Vintage, 1999); Jael Silliman and Marlene Gerber Fried, eds., *Undivided Rights: Women of Color Organizing for Reproductive Justice* (Chicago: Haymarket Books, 2016); Loretta Ross and Rickie Solinger, *Reproductive Justice: An Introduction* (Berkeley: University of California Press, 2017); Julia Oparah and Alicia Bonaparte, eds., *Birthing Justice: Black Women, Pregnancy, and Childbirth* (Abingdon: Routledge, 2015).
5. I'm inspired here by the findings of two important historians: Judith Leavitt, who notes in the introduction of *Brought to Bed* how she had been "struck more often by the congruence of [women's and physicians accounts of childbirth] than by their divergence" (9),

and Susan Reverby, who in *Examining Tuskegee* very successfully unravels the multiple meanings and memories of Tuskegee from the actual experiences on the ground. See Judith Walzer Leavitt, *Brought to Bed: Childbearing in America, 1750–1950* (New York: Oxford University Press, 2016); Susan Reverby, *Examining Tuskegee: The Infamous Syphilis Study and Its Legacy* (Chapel Hill: University of North Carolina Press, 2009).

6. Linda Bennett, interview with author, September 27, 2014.
7. Katy Butler, "Women: Midwifery on Trial in Santa Cruz," *San Francisco Bay Guardian*, July 20, 1974.
8. Ibid.
9. Linda Bennett, interview with author, September 27, 2014.
10. Eliza Avellar, nursing consultant for the family health services section of the State Department of Public Health, cited in Kaye Yost, "At Home or in the Hospital?" *San Francisco Examiner and Chronicle* November 3, 1974.
11. Raven Lang, *Birth Book* (1972; repr., Felton, CA: Genesis Press, 2007), 2.
12. Kate Bowland, "I Never Intended to Be an Outlaw," in Geradine Simkins, ed. *Into These Hands: Wisdom from Midwives* (Traverse City, MI: Spirituality and Health Books, 2011), 74.
13. Barbara Zheutlin and David Talbot, "California vs. Midwives: The Legalities of Attending a Birth," *Rolling Stone*, May 23, 1974, pp. 12–13.
14. Kenyon Jordan, "Pregnant State Agent Sets Up Birth Center," *Santa Cruz Times*, March 14, 1974.
15. Linda Bennett, interview with author, September 27, 2014.
16. Raven Lang, email correspondence with author, January 25, 2015.
17. Santa Cruz Birth Center to "friends," March 7, 1974, Kate Bowland personal collection.
18. Lang, email correspondence with author, January 25, 2015.
19. Ibid.
20. Raven Lang quoted in "The Art of Midwifery, Part II," *The Doula: A Magazine for Mothers*, 1 (4) Spring/Summer 1986, p. 2.
21. Raven Lang, interview with author, August 12, 2011.
22. Lang quoted in "The Art of Midwifery," *Doula*, p. 3.
23. Ibid.
24. Raven Lang, interview with author, August 12, 2011.
25. Lang quoted in "The Art of Midwifery," *Doula*, p. 3.
26. Raven Lang, interview with author, August 12, 2011.
27. Lay midwives were midwives who had not participated in a credentialed midwifery program. In the early 1990s, most lay midwives opted to identify themselves as "direct-entry midwives" in order to "emphasize both their professional competence and their unique point of entry into midwifery." See Christine Barbara Johnson, "Creating a Way out of No Way: Midwifery in Massachusetts," in *Mainstreaming Midwives: The Politics of Change*, Robbie Davis-Floyd and Christine Barbara Johnson, eds. (New York: Routledge, 2006), 375–410, quotation on 393. I have chosen to use the term *lay midwife* because that is how they commonly referred to themselves in the 1970s.
28. Lang quoted in "The Art of Midwifery," *Doula*, p. 4.
29. Raven Lang, interview with author, August 12, 2011.
30. Suzanne Arms, *Immaculate Deception: A New Look at Women and Childbirth in America* (Boston: Houghton Mifflin, 1975), 204.
31. Raven Lang, interview with author, August 12, 2011.
32. Lang quoted in "The Art of Midwifery," *Doula*, p. 5.
33. Ibid.
34. See Wendy Kline, *Bodies of Knowledge: Sexuality, Reproduction, and Women's Health in the Second Wave* (Chicago: University of Chicago Press, 2010), ch. 1.

35. Robert S. Spitzer, *Tidings of Comfort and Joy: An Anthology of Change* (Palo Alto: Science and Behavior Books, Inc., 1975), 219.
36. Arms, *Immaculate Deception*, 211.
37. In her study of nurse-midwife Ruth Watson Lubic, Julie Fairman notes the negative reaction of many obstetricians to out-of-hospital births in New York City in the mid-1970s, due to "competition and conflict." See Julie Fairman, "'Go to Ruth's House': The Social Activism of Ruth Lubic and the Family Health and Birth Center," *Nursing History Review* 18 (2010): 118–129, 121.
38. Arms, *Immaculate Deception*, 211.
39. Lang, *Birth Book*, 3.
40. Ibid.
41. Arms, *Immaculate Deception*, 212.
42. Lang, *Birth Book*, 152.
43. Ibid., 3.
44. Arms, *Immaculate Deception*.
45. Raven Lang, interview with author, August 12, 2011.
46. Linda Sibley, Elena Sibley, quoted in Lang, *Birth Book*, 120–122.
47. Lang, *Birth Book*, 126
48. Ibid., 130.
49. Ibid., 4.
50. "Childbirth at Home: A Seminar with the Santa Cruz Birth Center," flier, Bowland's personal collection. Italics added.
51. Lang, *Birth Book*, 150.
52. Ibid., 154–56.
53. This is a topic that Barbara Katz Rothman drew attention to early on, in her book, *In Labor*. "Many feminists became involved with women's health issues through organizing around abortion, where the right of women to control their own bodies was being denied by the state," she argues. "It was women organizing around the issue of abortion who began to raise questions about medical expansion into ethical concerns, bringing essentially moral issues under medical control." See Rothman, *In Labor: Women and Power in the Birthplace* (New York: W. W. Norton, 1991), 96, 109.
54. Linda Bennett, interview with author, September 27, 2014.
55. Ibid.
56. http://www.ppactionca.org/issues/abortion.html.
57. Linda Bennett, interview with author, September 27, 2014.
58. Ibid.
59. Ibid.
60. Sarah Abigail Leavitt, "'A Private Little Revolution': The Home Pregnancy Test in American Culture," *Bulletin of the History of Medicine*, 80 (2), Summer 2006, 326–27.
61. Leavitt, "A Private Little Revolution," 323.
62. Linda Bennett, interview with author, September 27, 2014.
63. Ibid.
64. Ibid.
65. For more on heightened consumer expectations, see Nancy Tomes, *Remaking the American Patient*, ch. 9.
66. Linda Bennett, interview with author, September 27, 2014.
67. Bowland, "I Never Intended," *Into These Hands*, 68.
68. Robin Imlay, "An Interview with Kate Bowland," May 5, 1987 (unpublished), Kate Bowland personal collection, p. 1.
69. Bowland, "I Never Intended," *Into These Hands*, 66.

70. "Impact Productions Presents PUSH: A WOMEN'S WESTERN," Press Release, ND, Kate Bowland personal collection.

71. Imlay, "An Interview with Kate Bowland," p. 2.

72. Judith Walzer Leavitt's article, "'Strange Young Women on Errands': Obstetric Nursing between Two Worlds" in *Nursing History Review* 6 (1998): 3–24, analyzes the role of gender and expectations of comfort and care in the maternity ward from the 1930s through the 1950s. Bowland's journal entry hints that these assumptions continued into the 1970s, and that the conflicts between nurses and midwives centered not only on training and expertise, but also on gendered expectations. See also Wendy Simonds, "Women in White," in Simonds and Rothman, *Laboring On: Birth in Transition in the United States* (New York: Routledge, 2006). Simonds writes, "Nurses clearly saw their jobs as involving the negotiation of a system in which they wielded little power. Four of the five nurses we interviewed told of their difficulties navigating the standard medical protocols and doctors' demands in ways that were similar to those of the midwives, but they had .. less clout and less autonomy than midwives. Most resented their disadvantaged status in the hospital hierarchy" (230).

73. Jay and Saxson discussed this in an unpublished interview with Jackie Christeve, Kate Bowland personal collection.

74. Kate Bowland, journal entry, ND, Bowland personal collection.

75. Linda Bennett, interview with author, September 27, 2014.

76. Katy Butler, "Women: Midwifery on Trial in Santa Cruz," *San Francisco Bay Guardian*, July 20, 1974.

77. Kate Bowland, journal entry, April 21, 1973, Bowland personal collection.

78. Kate Bowland, journal entry, March 21, 1973, Bowland personal collection.

79. Jeffrey J. Kripal, *Esalen: America and the Religion of No Religion* (Chicago: University of Chicago Press, 2007), 257.

80. Jean Mercer, *Alternative Psychotherapies: Evaluating Mental Health Treatments* (Lanham, MD: Rowman and Littlefield, 2014), 114.

81. Kate Bowland, journal entry, March 21, 1973, Bowland personal collection.

82. Ibid.

83. Ibid.

84. Kate Bowland, journal entry, April 21, 1973, Bowland personal collection.

85. Kate Bowland, journal entry, ND, Bowland personal collection.

86. Kate Bowland, speaking in *PUSH* documentary.

87. http://www.usclimatedata.com/climate/santa-cruz/california/united-states/usca1020.

88. Jeffrey J. Kripal, *Esalen: America and the Religion of No Religion* (Chicago: University of Chicago Press, 2007), 258.

89. Raven Lang, email correspondence with author, January 25, 2015.

90. Bowland, "I Never Intended," 72.

91. Kate Bowland, journal entry, ND, Bowland personal collection.

92. Ultimately Cumings tried to challenge the constitutionality of the law, arguing it was "vague" and "overbroad."

93. Linda Bennett, interview with author, September 27, 2014.

94. Tom Honig, "Midwives' Petition Denied; Appeal Vowed," *Santa Cruz Sentinel*, September 1, 1974, p. 37.

95. https://www.dshs.state.tx.us/midwife/mw_history.shtm.

96. "Midwives Lose a Legal Round," *Santa Cruz Sentinel*, August 18, 1974, p. 29.

97. For more on fetal personhood, see Sara Dubow, *Ourselves Unborn: A History of the Fetus in Modern America* (New York: Oxford University Press, 2010).

98. Katy Butler, "Women: Midwifery on Trial in Santa Cruz," *San Francisco Bay Guardian*, July 20, 1974.

99. Babara Zheutlin and David Talbot, "California vs. Midwives: The Legalities of Attending a Birth," *Rolling Stone*, May 23, 1974, pp. 12–13.

100. Cumings, "Appellant's Opening Brief," *Bowland v. Municipal Court of Santa Cruz County Judicial District*, 1/Civil No. 35739, Ehrlich personal collection.

101. According to Raymond DeVries, there were only approximately 170 certified nurse-midwives practicing in California in 1981, and most of these working in large metropolitan hospitals. See DeVries, *Making Midwives Legal: Childbirth, Medicine, and the Law*, 2nd ed. (Columbus: Ohio State University Press, 1996), 71.

102. ACLU statement quoted in "Respondent's Brief: Appeal from the Judgment of the Superior Court of the State of California for the County of Santa Cruz," *Bowland v. Municipal Court of Santa Cruz County Judicial District*, 1/Civil No. 35739, p. 21, Bowland personal collection.

103. In *Laboring On*, Wendy Simonds points out the "irony in the midwifery community's use of 'choice', because abortion is a potentially divisive issue within that community. There are midwives who are profoundly pro-choice, who have come to midwifery and their pro-choice positions out of the same commitment to women, out of a vision of feminism" (197).

104. As scholar Mary Lay argues, though *Roe* "appeared to expand women's reproductive choices and control over their own bodies," in some instances it did the reverse. Mary Lay, *The Rhetoric of Midwifery: Gender, Knowledge, and Power* (Rutgers, 2000), 60.

105. Linda Bennett, interview with author, September 27, 2014.

106. Cumings and Jordan, "Appellant's Closing Brief," May 12, 1975," *Bowland v. Municipal Court of Santa Cruz County Judicial District*, 1/Civil No. 35739, p. 9, Bowland personal collection.

107. Cumings, "Petition for Rehearing," December 20, 1976, *Bowland v. Municipal Court of Santa Cruz County Judicial District*, No. S.F. 23484 In the Supreme Court of the State of California, p. 6, Karen Ehrlich personal collection.

108. For a valuable legal analysis on the impact of *Bowland* on other state decisions, (in MA, CO, and NJ) see Michael A. Pike, "Restriction of Parental Rights to Home Births Via State Regulation of Traditional Midwifery," *Brandeis Journal of Family Law*, Fall, 1997. Pike notes that the resulting judicial decisions "produce odd practical results which state legislatures and courts most likely did not foresee when they drafted and interpreted midwifery statutes." He notes that they "might convince both ardent Roe v Wade and abortion opponents and abortion supporters that in many ways *Roe* actually went too far in giving the State power over the health and safety of women and children." (611).

109. Though the increasing number of forced C-sections beginning in the 1980s suggests that both midwives and laboring women are now legal targets.

110. Though of course that reasoning was somewhat faulty, as many have chosen unassisted childbirth rather than hospital birth. See Rixa Freeze, "Born Free: Unassisted Childbirth in North America," PhD dissertation, University of Iowa, 2008.

111. Santa Cruz Women's Health Collective, "Whatever Happened to Clinics? An Update from the Women's Health Collective," February 1976, p. 2, Bowland personal collection.

112. See Rebecca Kluchin, *Fit to Be Tied: Sterilization and Reproductive Rights in America, 1950–1980* (New Brunswick: Rutgers University Press, 2011); Jeanne Flavin, *Our Bodies, Our Crimes: The Policing of Women's Reproduction in America* (New York: New York University Press, 2010).

113. Kate Bowland, quoted in Robin Imlay, "An Interview with Kate Bowland," May 5, 1987 (unpublished), Kate Bowland personal collection, p. 3.

114. Sharon Steiner quoted in "First Day Discussions—Santa Cruz Midwives," September 1975, p. 10.

115. Ibid., p. 94.

116. Karen Ehrlich, "The Santa Cruz Birth Center Today," *Birth and the Family Journal*, 1976, p. 125.

117. Sharon Hamilton, "First Day Discussions," 65.

118. Kristen Thomas, "First Day Discussions," 74.

119. Kate Bowland conversation with author, July 15, 2011.

120. Mary Lay, "Midwifery on Trial: Balancing Privacy Rights and Health Concerns after Roe v. Wade," *Quarterly Journal of Speech*, 89:1, 60–77, 2003; Michael A. Pike, "Restriction of Parental Rights to Home Births Via State Regulation of Traditional Midwifery," *Brandeis Journal of Family Law*, Fall, 1997; Charles Wolfson, "Midwives and Home Birth: Social, Medical, and Legal Perspectives," *Hastings Law Journal* (37), May 1986; Amy Cohen, "The Midwifery Stalemate and Childbirth Choices: Recognizing Mothers-to-Be as the Best Decisionmakers," *Indiana Law Journal* (80): 849, Summer, 2005; Cynthia Watchorn, "Midwifery; A History of Statutory Suppression," *Golden Gate University Law Review* vol. 9, issue 2, 1978; Julie Harmon, "Statutory Regulations of Midwives: A Study of California Law," *William and Mary Journal of Women and the Law*, vol. 8 issue 1 (2001): 115–132; David M. Smolin, "The Jurisprudence of Privacy in a Splintered Supreme Court," *Marquette Law Review* (75): 975 (Summer, 1992).

CHAPTER 5

1. https://www.youtube.com/watch?v=iIl6VnjQjJ8.

2. https://mana.org/pdfs/MANA-E-zine-March-2014.pdf.

3. https://www.youtube.com/watch?v=iIl6VnjQjJ8.

4. http://www.hotelpdn.com/

5. Aryln MacDonald, "Impressions," *Mothering Magazine* Vol. 3, 1977 p. 52.

6. Carol Leonard, *Lady's Hands, Lion's Heart: A Midwife's Saga* (Hopkinton: Bad Beaver Press, 2008), 83.

7. Ibid.

8. Aryln MacDonald, "Impressions," 52.

9. Fran Ventre, "Recollections and Reflections on the Conference," *News from H.O.M.E*, Vol. 2 No. 1 (Winter 1977): 2. Fran Ventre Papers, 1970–2000; MC 772, Folder 8.2. Schlesinger Library, Radcliffe Institute, Harvard University, Cambridge, MA.

10. Marion Sousa, "Midwives Meet," *News from H.O.M.E.*, Vol. 2 No. 1 (Winter 1977): 1, Ventre Papers, Folder 8.2.

11. Leonard, *Lady's Hands, Lion's Heart*, 84.

12. Cumings quoted in *The Practicing Midwife* (1), p. 3, ND, Karen Ehrlich personal collection.

13. Hilary Schlinger, *Circle of Midwives: Organized Midwifery in North America* (self-pub., 1992), 6.

14. Karen Ehrlich, interview with author, August 6, 2011.

15. Nancy Tomes, *Remaking the American Patient: How Madison Avenue and Modern Medicine Turned Patients into Consumers* (Chapel Hill: University of North Carolina Press, 2016), 289.

16. Ibid., 299.

17. "At its peak, NAPSAC had more than 8,000 members for which the Stewarts wrote and published a newsletter, *The NAPSAC News*, with issues continuing over a twenty-year span, into the 1990's. Since the early 1970's, they have been among the early pioneers and international leaders in the promotion of home birth and breastfeeding." See http://www.raindroptraining.com/care/stewart.shtml.

18. Nancy Tomes, *Remaking the American Patient*, 6.

19. See, for example, Tomes, *Remaking the American Patient*; Susan Reverby, *Examining Tuskegee: The Infamous Syphilis Study and Its Legacy* (Chapel Hill: University of North

Carolina Press, 2009); David Rothman, *Strangers at the Bedside: A History of How Law and Bioethics Transformed Medical Decision Making* (New York: Basic Books, 1992).

20. "Merry May 1976," report to LLL Board of Directors, Box 87, La Leche League International Records (LLLI), DePaul University Archives, Chicago, IL.
21. Tomes, *Remaking the American Patient*, 266.
22. Schlinger, *Circle of Midwives*, 6.
23. Fran Ventre, "The Lay Midwife," originally presented at a workshop entitled "Partners for Health," sponsored by Chapter 6 of the ACNM on October 2, 1976. Reprinted in the *Journal of Nurse-Midwifery* 22, no. 4 (Winter 1978): 33.
24. Fran Ventre, email correspondence with author, December 13, 2011.
25. Ventre, *News from H.O.M.E.* vol. 1 no. 3, (Summer 1976): 4, Folder 8.2, Ventre papers.
26. Birthcenter midwives [exact location unknown] to El Paso conference coordinators, ND, Folder 6.5, Ventre papers. This argument would become central to the midwifery movement over the next few decades, first formally articulated in 1979 by Barbara Katz Rothman in her first book, *In Labor: Women and Power in the Birthplace*. The medical model of birth, promoted in hospitals and dictated by doctors, appeared antithetical to a midwifery model (In 1992, anthropologist Robbie Davis-Floyd labeled the two approaches a technocratic vs. a holistic model).
27. Carol Weisman, *Women's Health Care: Activist Traditions and Institutional Change* (Baltimore: Johns Hopkins University Press, 1998), 72.
28. First International Conference brochure, Kate Bowland personal collection.
29. "MIDWIFE STUDY GROUP" notes, November 22, 1976, Karen Ehrlich personal collection.
30. Allee Jay to Shari Daniels, November 26, 1976, Folder 6.5, Ventre papers. The letter is also signed by Santa Cruz midwives Karen Ehrlich and Kate Bowland.
31. Ibid.
32. Shari Daniels, 21 December 1976, Bowland personal collection.
33. Birthcenter midwives to El Paso conference coordinators, ND, Folder 6.5, Ventre papers.
34. Allee Jay to Shari Daniels, November 26, 1976, Ventre papers.
35. Fran Ventre to Allee Jay, Karen Ehrlich, and Kate Bowland, December 4, 1976, Bowland personal collection.
36. Shari Daniels to Allee Jay, December 21, 1976, Bowland personal collection.
37. Birthcenter midwives to El Paso conference coordinators, ND.
38. *The Practicing Midwife* (1), p. 2, ND, Karen Ehrlich personal collection.
39. Carson et al, "A Working Lay Midwife Home Birth Program in Seattle, Washington: A Collective Approach" (1977), pp 507–44 in Stewart and Stewart, eds., *21st Century Obstetrics Now!*, quoted in DeVries, *Making Midwives Legal: Childbirth, Medicine, and the Law* (Columbus: Ohio State University Press, 1996), 151–52.
40. Devries, *Making Midwives Legal*, 140.
41. Schlinger, *Circle of Midwives*, 10.
42. Aryln MacDonald, "Impressions," *Mothering* Magazine vol. 3 (1977): 54.
43. Karen Ehrlich, email correspondence with author, September 8, 2012.
44. Fran Ventre, "Recollections and Reflections on the Conference," *News from H.O.M.E.*, Vol 2. No. 1 p. 3.
45. Carol Leonard, *Lady's Hands, Lion's Heart*, 85.
46. Jill Frawley, *Mothering* Magazine, vol. 3 (1977).
47. Warren H. Pearse, MD, "Home Birth Crisis," ACOG Newsletter (July 1977), ACOG library, Washington, D.C.
48. Rahima Baldwin, *Special Delivery: The Choices are Yours* (Berkeley: Celestial Arts, 1979), 1.
49. Schlinger, *Circle of Midwives*, 6.

50. Winifred Connerton and Patricia D'Antonio, "International Comparisons: The Nursing-Midwifery Interface," in Anne Borsay and Billie Hunter, eds., *Nursing and Midwifery in Britain since 1700* (Basingstoke: Palgrave 2012), p. 190.

51. Judith Rooks, *Midwifery and Childbirth in America* (Philadelphia: Temple University Press, 1997), 66.

52. Ibid., 70–71.

53. ACNM Executive Board Meeting October 27, 1973. ACNM records, MSC 330a (37), National Library of Medicine, Bethesda, MD.

54. Ibid.

55. Helen Varney and Joyce Beebe Thompson, *The Midwife Said Fear Not: A History of Midwifery in the United States* (New York: Springer, 2016), 192.

56. Susan Leibel to ACNM Colleagues, September 5, 1977, ACNM records, MSC 330a (11.24).

57. Susan Leibel to Carmela, Sept 5, 1977, ACNM records, MSC 330a (11.24).

58. Susan Leibel-Finkle, quoted in Hillary Schlinger, *Circle of Midwives*, 8–9.

59. Though of course the earlier home birth statement controversy stemmed from this movement.

60. Susan Leibel to ACNM Colleagues, December 28, 1977, ACNM records, MSC 330a (11.24).

61. Susan Leibel to ACNM Colleagues, March 20, 1978, ACNM records, MSC 330a (11.24).

62. Lang quoted in Schlinger, *Circle of Midwives*, 11.

63. Ibid., 11–12.

64. Sister Angela Murdaugh quoted in Schlinger, *Circle of Midwives*, 15.

65. Murdaugh mentions this in August 24 1981 memo to Special Presidential Task Force on Dialogue with Lay Midwives; letter and check arrived from ABCC on Sept 29, 1981. ACNM records, MSC 330a (5.11).

66. Murdaugh to Ina May Gaskin August 24, 1981, ACNM records, MSC 330a (5.11).

67. Gaskin to Murdaugh, 27 August 1981, ACNM records, MSC 330a (5.11).

68. Murdaugh explains in a memo dated August 24 1981 to the Special Presidential Task Force on Dialogue with Lay Midwives that she also telephoned Helen Marieskind from the Seattle Midwifery School, but that Marieskind would not be able to attend the meeting. At a later date, Teddy Charvet (who later changed her name to Therese Stallings) was sent as the SMS representative.

69. Helen Jolly to Murdaugh, August 28, 1981, ACNM records, MSC 330a (5.11).

70. Elisabeth Blish Genly to Murdaugh, October 3, 1981, ACNM records, MSC 330a (5.11).

71. Murdaugh to ACNM members, November 18, 1981, ACNM records, MSC 330a (5.11).

72. See Jennifer Nelson, *More than Medicine: A History of the Feminist Women's Health Movement* (New York: New York University Press, 2015), 16. Nelson argues that many women's health activists' initial involvement in activism was in the civil rights and student movements of the 1960s.

73. Murdaugh to ACNM members, November 18, 1981, ACNM records, MSC 330a (5.11).

74. Charvet quoted in Schlinger, *Circle of Midwives*, 16.

75. Cumings quoted in *The Practicing Midwife* (1), p. 3, ND, Karen Ehrlich personal collection.

76. Murdaugh to ACNM members, November 18, 1981, ACNM records, MSC 330a (5.11).

77. Genna Withrow to Fran Ventre, Ina May Gaskin, Carol Hurzeler, Susan Leibel, Helen Jolly, and Teddy Charvet, November 20, 1981, Box 1 Folder 2, Midwives Alliance of North America Records, MS 375, Sophia Smith Collection, Smith College, Northampton, Mass.

78. Carol Hurzeler to Ina May Gaskin, January 28, 1982, Box 1 Folder 2, Midwives Alliance of North America Records.

79. Ibid.

80. Ina May Gaskin to Susan Leibel, February 4, 1982, Box 1 Folder 2, Midwives Alliance of North America Records.

81. Teddy Charvet, February 2, 1982, Box 1 Folder 2, Midwives Alliance of North America Records.

82. Ina May Gaskin to Susan Leibel, Carol Hurzeler, Helen Jolly, Genna Withrow, Fran Ventre, and Teddy Charvet, February 16, 1982. Box 1 Folder 2, Midwives Alliance of North America Records.

83. Marion Donahue, audio cassette recording of MANA meeting, April 24, 1982, Carol Leonard personal collection.

84. Linda Cozzolino, audio cassette recording of MANA meeting, April 24, 1982.

85. Ina May Gaskin to Farm midwives Cara, Mary, Gerrie Sue, and Kay Marie, May 3, 1982, p. 2. Box 1 Folder 2, Midwives Alliance of North America Records.

86. Susan Leibel, audio cassette recording of MANA meeting, April 24, 1982.

87. Marion Donahue, audio cassette recording of MANA meeting, April 24, 1982.

88. Linda Cozzolino, audio cassette recording of MANA meeting, April 24, 1982.

89. Ibid.

90. Ruth Beanham, audio cassette recording of MANA meeting, April 24, 1982.

91. Ibid.

92. Dorothy Richards, audio cassette recording of MANA meeting, April 24, 1982.

93. Ina May Gaskin, audio cassette recording of MANA meeting, April 24, 1982.

94. Susan Leibel, audio cassette recording of MANA meeting, April 24, 1982.

95. Linda Irene-Green, audio cassette recording of MANA meeting, April 24, 1982.

96. Ibid.

97. Kate Newson, audio cassette recording of MANA meeting, April 24, 1982.

98. Ina May Gaskin to Farm midwives Cara, Mary, Gerrie Sue, and Kay Marie, May 3, 1982, p. 7. Box 1 Folder 2, Midwives Alliance of North America Records.

99. Susan Leibel, audio cassette recording of MANA meeting, April 24, 1982.

100. Ina May Gaskin to Farm midwives Cara, Mary, Gerrie Sue, and Kay Marie, May 3, 1982, p. 8. Box 1 Folder 2, Midwives Alliance of North America Records.

101. Ibid., p. 9.

102. Ibid.

103. Susan Leibel to Ms. Vogler, June 9, 1982, Box 1 Folder 2, Midwives Alliance of North America Records.

104. Susan Leibel to Colleagues, June 9, 1982, Box 1 Folder 2, Midwives Alliance of North America Records.

105. Beatrice Carline to Ina May Gaskin, July 23, 1982, Box 15 Folder 1, Midwives Alliance of North America Records.

106. Lea Rizack to Ina May Gaskin, Feb 18, 1983, Box 15 Folder 1, Midwives Alliance of North America Records.

107. Lani Rosenberger to Ina May Gaskin (who retypes and forwards to Teddy and Carol, 25 February, 1985), Box 15 Folder 1, Midwives Alliance of North America Records.

108. Teddy Charvet to Lani Rosenberger, Mar 29, 1985, Box 15 Folder 1, Midwives Alliance of North America Records.

109. Anne Frye to Ina May Gaskin, June 19, 1983, Box 18 Folder 1, Midwives Alliance of North America Records.

110. Susan Leibel to Anne Frye, July 24, 1983, Box 16 Folder 3, Midwives Alliance of North America Records.

111. Teddy Charvet to Anne Frye, July 18, 1983, Box 15 Folder 2, Midwives Alliance of North America Records.

112. Ruth Harvey and Lillian Anderson to MANA, December 19, 1990, Box 6 Folder 3, Midwives Alliance of North America Records.

113. Julia Chinyere Oparah with Black Women Birthing Justice, "Beyond Coercion and Malign Neglect: Black Women and the Struggle for Birth Justice," in *Birthing Justice: Black Women, Pregnancy, and Childbirth* (Routledge, 2016), p. 14.

114. Ruth Harvey and Lillian Anderson to MANA, December 19, 1990.

115. Minutes of the MANA board of directors meeting, New Orleans, October 25–27, 1988, p. 6, Box 12 Folder 7, Midwives Alliance of North America Records.

116. Sharon Ransom in MANA News, Vol 7 No. 3, Sept. 1989, quoted in Schlinger, *Circle of Midwives*, 75.

117. Sondra Abdullah Zaimah, quoted in Schlinger, *Circle of Midwives*, 75.

CHAPTER 6

1. Ivan Illich, *Medical Nemisis: The Expropriation of Health* (New York: Random House, 1976), 3–6.

2. Nancy Tomes, *Remaking the American Patient*, 257.

3. Carson, Felton, Gloyd, Luehrs, Mansfield, Mertz, Myers, Rivard (Fremont Women's Clinic/Birth Collective), "A Working Lay Midwife Home Birth Program," *21st Century Obstetrics Now!* Vol. 2, p. 519. As Nancy Tomes notes, health care became a way for activist groups to "broaden their base of support within the larger community." Tomes, *Remaking the American Patient*, 257.

4. Carson et al., "A Working Lay Midwife Home Birth Program," *21st Century Obstetrics Now!* p. 520.

5. Suzy Myers, interview with author, July 21, 2015.

6. Jennifer Nelson, *More than Medicine: A History of the Feminist Women's Health Movement* (New York: NYU Press, 2015), 97.

7. John Dittmer, *The Good Doctors: The Medical Committee for Human Rights and the Struggle for Social Justice in Health Care* (London: Bloomsbury Press, 2009), 223.

8. Nelson, *More than Medicine*, 100.

9. Jo Anne Myers-Ciecko, interview with author, July 22, 2015.

10. Jo Anne Myers-Ciecko, interview with Beth Coyote, May 11, 1999, Beth Coyote personal collection.

11. Marge Mansfield, interview with Beth Coyote, May 18, 1999, Coyote personal collection.

12. See Nelson, *More than Medicine*, 95, 93.

13. Ibid., 117.

14. Ibid., 96.

15. Ibid., 100.

16. Mansfield, interview with Beth Coyote, May 18, 1999, Coyote personal collection.

17. Judi Modie, "Babies Born at Home," *Seattle Post-Intelligencer*, 1971 [ND, first in series of 4], Folder "Articles/News Clippings 1971–77," Box 17, Seattle Midwifery School records, 1978–2009 [Hereafter SMS records], Collection number 5597, University of Washington Libraries, Special Collections, Seattle, WA.

18. Jo Anne Myers-Ciecko, "Midwifery in the United States," in Sheila Kitzinger, ed., *The Midwife Challenge*, edited by Sheila Kitzinger," SMS records Box 17 p. 22.

19. Judi Hunt, "Home Deliveries Aren't Just a Fad," *Seattle Post-Intelligencer*, June 28, 1976, p. A-8, SMS records, Folder "Articles/News Clippings 1971-77," Box 17.

20. Grace M. Jansons, "Synopsis of Report Submitted to the October 1 Meeting of the WSMC re: growth in demand for home births," SMS records, Folder "Legislation WSMC77-79," Box 17.

21. Myers interview with author, July 21, 2015.

22. Carson et al., "A Working Lay Midwife Home Birth Program," 509.

23. Myers interview with author, July 21, 2015.

24. Marge Mansfield, interview with Beth Coyote, May 18, 1999, Coyote personal collection.

25. Myers interview with author, July 21, 2015.

26. Carson et al., "A Working Lay Midwife Home Birth Program," 509.

27. Ibid., 510.

28. Myers interview with author, July 21, 2015.

29. Ibid.

30. Carson et al., "A Working Lay Midwife Home Birth Program," 510–511.

31. Ibid., 524.

32. See Judith A. Houck, "The Best Prescription for Women's Health: Feminist Approaches to Well-Woman Care," in Jeremy Greene and Elizabeth Watkins, *Prescribed: Writing, Filling, Using, and Abusing the Prescription in Modern America* (Johns Hopkins University Press, 2012), pp. 134–56; Nelson, *More than Medicine.*

33. Carson et al., "A Working Lay Midwife Home Birth Program," 508.

34. Ibid.; Nelson, *More than Medicine*, 99.

35. Carson et al., "A Working Lay Midwife Home Birth Program," NAPSAC, 522.

36. A background in civil rights and new New left Left organizations was common for women's health activists, as Jennifer Nelson demonstrates in *More than Medicine.*

37. Suzy Myers, interview with author, July 21, 2015.

38. Nelson, *More than Medicine*, 2.

39. Jo Anne Myers-Ciecko, interview with Beth Coyote, May 11, 1999, Coyote personal collection.

40. Jo Anne Myers-Ciecko, interview with author, July 21, 2015.

41. Jo Anne Myers-Ciecko, interview with Beth Coyote, May 11, 1999, Coyote personal collection.

42. Suzy Myers, interview with author, July 21, 2015.

43. Marge Mansfield, interview with Beth Coyote, May 18, 1999, Coyote personal collection.

44. S.B. Thacker and H.D. Banta, "Benefits and risks of episiotomy: an interpretative review of the English language literature, 1860–1980." *Obstetrical & Gynecological Survey* (1983 June) 38(6): 322–338.

45. R.J. Woolley, "Benefits and risks of episiotomy: a review of the English-language literature since 1980." Part I. *Obstetrical & Gynecological Survey* (1995 November) 50(11): 806–820.

46. Suzy Myers, interview with author, July 21, 2015.

47. Marge Mansfield, interview with Beth Coyote, May 18, 1999, Coyote personal collection.

48. Carson et al., "A Working Lay Midwife Home Birth Program," 513.

49. See Nancy Tomes, *Remaking the American Patient*, ch. 8.

50. Ruth S. Anderson, Administrative Nursing Supervisor, "Guidelines Regarding Patients from the Fremont Clinic," Interdepartmental memo, December 10, 1975, Beth Coyote personal collection.

51. In chapter 6 of *Make Room for Daddy: The Journey from Waiting Room to Birthing Room* (Chapel Hill: University of North Carolina Press, 2010), 195–235, Judith Walzer Leavitt describes hospital resistance to (and ultimate success of) fathers' access to delivery rooms, noting multiple reasons for the rigid hospital policies of exclusion. Among these were privacy (men's presence could interfere with privacy of other patients) interference, and safety.

52. Zane Brown, MD, to Fremont Women's Clinic, December 22, 1977, Box 14, Folder "Founding Documents, 1977," SMS records. For more on how hospitals changed hospital delivery wards to accommodate the demands of patients (and fathers), see Judith Leavitt, *Make Room for Daddy.*

53. As sociologist Wendy Simonds notes, "You can domesticate the surroundings by hanging floral wallpaper and providing padded rocking chairs. But redecorating will not alter

conventional power dynamics, as long as the precepts of obstetrical monitoring remain in place and the operating room is right down the hall from the labor and delivery 'suites.' " Wendy Simonds, Barbara Katz Rothman, and Bari Meltzer Norman, *Laboring On: Birth in Transition in the United States* (Abingdon: Routledge, 2006), 192.

54. Zane Brown, MD, to Fremont Women's Clinic, December 22, 1977, SMS Box 14, Folder "Founding Documents, 1977."

55. Sherry Taber to Mr. James W. Varnum, Hospital Administrator, November 17, 1977, Coyote personal collection.

56. Ibid.

57. Fremont Women's Clinic Birth Collective to Dennis Scholl, Director, Ultrasound Department, University Hospital, February 2, 1978, Coyote personal collection.

58. Dennis G. School MD, to Fremont Women's Clinic, February 24, 1978, Coyote personal collection.

59. Angela Bowen, MD, Chairman, to Martha Butzen, October 1, 1976, Coyote personal collection.

60. Angela Bowen, MD, letter to Tom Artzner, October 1, 1976, Coyote personal collection.

61. Carson et al., "A Working Lay Midwife Home Birth Program," 520–521.

62. Fremont Women's Birth Collective to clients, June 15, 1977, Coyote personal collection.

63. Myers, interview with author, July 21, 2015.

64. Marge Mansfield, interview with Beth Coyote, May 18, 1999, Coyote personal collection.

65. Suzy Myers' PowerPoint presentation, 2010 graduation, Myers personal collection.

66. Marge Mansfield, interview with Beth Coyote, May 18, 1999, Coyote personal collection.

67. http://seattlemedium.com/dr-r-y-roz-woodhouse/.

68. http://www.historylink.org/File/8470.

69. Fremont Women's Clinic to Ms. R. Woodhouse, August 17, 1977, appendix I of 1979 Funding Proposal, SMS Box 14.

70. Seattle Midwifery School to friends, November 20, 1978, SMS Box 10, Folder "Development 1978–85."

71. Marge Mansfield, interview with Beth Coyote, May 18, 1999, Coyote personal collection.

72. Suzy Myers, interview with author, July 21, 2015.

73. Seattle Midwifery School to friends, November 20, 1978, SMS Box 10, Folder "Development 1978–85."

74. "Working Towards a Legal Midwifery Practice," p. 3, SMS Box 14, Folder "Founding Documents 1977."

75. Marge Mansfield, interview with Beth Coyote, May 18, 1999, Coyote personal collection.

76. Katherine Camacho Carr, "Evaluation of Proposed Curriculum for School of Midwifery," June 14, 1978, "Letters of Support for School to Div. of Prof. Lic.," Coyote personal collection.

77. It should be noted however, that this good will did not last; notes recorded in the "daily log" suggest that attempts to work with some of these CNMs on teaching and preceptorships did not end well.

78. Elaine P. Schurmann to Joan Baird, Administrator, Div. of Professional Licensing, June 29, 1978, "Letters of Support for School to Div. of Prof. Lic.," Coyote personal collection.

79. Rosemary Mann to Joan Baird, June 28, 1978, "Letters of Support for School to Div. of Prof. Lic.," Coyote personal collection.

80. George C. Hibbs to Joan Baird, June 29, 1979, "Letters of Support for School to Div. of Prof. Lic.," Coyote personal collection.

81. Philip D. DuBois to Joan Baird, August 1, 1978, "Letters of Support for School to Div. of Prof. Lic.," Coyote personal collection.

82. Philip D. DuBois to Joan Baird, August 1, 1978, "Letters of Support for School to Div. of Prof. Lic.," Coyote personal collection.

83. Marcia J. Colemen to Joan Baird, August 5, 1978, "Letters of Support for School to Div. of Prof. Lic.," Coyote personal collection.

84. On December 22, 1977, Brown wrote the Fremont Birth Collective thanking them for their support and good will. "If I can be of any help to you or your patients at any time in the future, please do not hesitate to call on me, day or night." SMS Box 14, Folder "Founding Documents, 1977."

85. Zane Brown to SMS, June 14, 1978, "Letters of Support for School to Div. of Prof. Lic.," Coyote personal collection.

86. Steve Gloyd to R.Y. Woodhouse, October 21, 1978, "Steve Gloyd's old notes on Seattle Midwifery School," Coyote personal collection.

87. Ibid.

88. Ibid.

89. Susan Anemone and James Mundt, "Proposal to Fund a Midwifery Training Program at the Seattle Midwifery School," March 1979, Box 141, Folder "SMS MEP Funding Proposal 1979," p. 2.

90. Ibid., p. 5.

91. Ibid., pp. 6–7.

92. The first group of students were Suzy Meyers, Susan Anemone, Suzi Rivard, and Marge Mansfield. Miriamma Carson, also from the Fremont Birth Collective, was the fifth student, but opted not to be involved in the administration of the school.

93. "First Meeting of Advisory Board and Board of Directors of Seattle Midwifery School," February 12, 1979, p. 3. SMS Box 15.

94. Suzy Myers, interview with author, July 21, 2015.

95. Marge Mansfield, interview with Beth Coyote, May 18, 1999, Coyote personal collection.

96. First Meeting of Advisory Board and Board of Directors of Seattle Midwifery School, February 12, 1979, p. 3. SMS Box 15.

97. Suzy Myers and Jo Anne Myers-Ciecko interview with author, July 22, 2015.

98. Ibid.

99. Marge Mansfield, interview with Beth Coyote, May 18, 1999, Coyote personal collection.

100. Suzy Myers, interview with author, July 21, 2015.

101. Daily log, March 25, 1980, Coyote personal collection.

102. Marge Mansfield, interview with Beth Coyote, May 18, 1999, Coyote personal collection.

103. Daily log, April 24, 1980, Coyote personal collection.

104. Suzy Myers' PowerPoint presentation at ACNM meeting, 2009, Myers personal collection.

105. Minutes of Advisory Board Meeting, February 21, 1980, p. 2., SMS Box 15, Folder "B of D 1979–1980."

106. Board of Directors meeting, October 13, 1983, SMS Box 15, Folder "B of D 1983."

107. SMS to students [draft], January 31, 1981, sent to Board Members, SMS Box 15, Folder "B of D 1981."

108. "Legislative Alert," January 18, 1980, SMS Box 17 Folder "Midwifery Legislation, 1979–80."

109. Letter to students [draft], January 31, 1981, sent to Board Members, SMS Box 15, B of D 1981.

110. Ibid.

111. Jo Anne Myers-Ciecko, interview with Beth Coyote, May 11, 1999, Coyote personal collection.

112. Suzy Myers to Jo Anne Myers-Ciecko, January 4, 1979, SMS Box 14, Folder "Founding Documents/Early Corresp 1979–80."

113. Scene Four, History of SMS Skit, SMS Box 14.

114. Jo Anne Myers-Ciecko, interview with Beth Coyote, May 11, 1999, Coyote personal collection.

115. Ibid.

116. Nancy Wainer Cohen, July 26, 1996 journal entry, Box 4, Folder 1, Nancy Wainer Cohen papers, MC 656, Schlesinger library, Harvard University, Cambridge, MA.

117. Advisory Board meeting, February 21, 1980, SMS Box 9, Folder "B of D 1979–80."

118. Board of Directors meeting, October 1, 1981, SMS Box 9, Folder "B of D 1981."

119. Board of Directors meeting, May 12, 1983, Box 9, Folder "B of D 1982–83."

120. As Sheryl Nestel points out, such limited options resulted in a proliferation of midwifery clinics on the U.S. –Mexico border. These clinics have for the last twenty years "been a significant training site for those unwilling or unable to pursue long and expensive apprenticeships in the few available programs. The clinics have been popular because they enable direct-entry midwifery students to attend large numbers of births within a relatively short time." See Nestel, *Obstructed Labor: Race and Gender in the Re-Emergence of Midwifery* (Vancouver: University of British Columbia Press, 2006), 76.

121. SMS Education Committee meeting, October 27, 1981, SMS Box 9, Folder "B of D 1981."

122. Education Committee meeting, January 25, 1982, SMS Box 9.

123. Seven of the midwives or midwifery students Nestel interviewed for her study had participated in midwifery tourism between 1978 and 1997. See Nestel, *Obstructed Labor,* p. 76.

124. Nestel, *Obstructed Labor,* 70.

125. Wendy Gordon, "Why ALL Midwives Should Care About What's Going On with Midwife International," September 4, 2013, *Aromidwifery.* https://aromidwifery.wordpress.com/2013/09/04/why-all-midwives-should-care-about-whats-going-on-with-midwife-international/.

126. Marge Mansfield to Percival McDonald, February 19, 1986, SMS Box 5, Folder "St. Lucia Correspondence file"; Russell, Gwynne, and Trisolini, "Health Care Financing in St. Lucia and Costs of Victoria Hospital," Research Report No. 5, Stoney Brook, NY, May 1988, 5–6.

127. http://stlucianheroes.com/sr-mary-irma-hilger/, http://www.stjudehospitalslu.org/.

128. Russell, Gwynne, and Trisolini, "Health Care Financing in St. Lucia and Costs of Victoria Hospital," p. 9.

129. Unfortunately, the actual letter is not in the archives; this issue only appears in the minutes of the SMS steering committee, and they do not reveal the nature of her complaints.

130. SMS Steering Committee Minutes, July 6, 1983, SMS Box 9.

131. Board of Directors Minutes, January 12 1984, SMS Box 9.

132. Board of Directors Minutes, November 30 1983, SMS Box 9.

133. Marge Mansfield to Matron Parker at Victoria Hospital, February 19, 1986, SMS Box 5, Folder "St. Lucia Correspondence 7/82-9/92."

134. Russell, Gwynne, and Trisolini, "Health Care Financing in St. Lucia and Costs of Victoria Hospital," p. 26.

135. Ibid., 10–11.

136. Ibid., 105.

137. Student postcard, postmarked June 15, 1987, SMS Box 5, Folder "St. Lucia '86–87."

138. Student postcard, November 2, 1987, SMS Box 5, Folder "St. Lucia 86–87."

139. Beth Coyote, interview with author, July 25, 2015.

140. Karen Hays and Sarah Huntington, "St. Lucia: Some Tips from Our Experience," SMS Box 5, Folder "St. Lucia Corresp 7/82–9/92."

141. Nestel, *Obstructed Labor,* p. 82.

142. K. Shaw, "Castries and Victoria Hospital Notes," October 1986, SMS Box 5, Folder "St. Lucia '86–87."

143. Karen Hays and Sarah Huntington, "St. Lucia: Some Tips from Our Experience," Box 5, Folder "St. Lucia Corresp 7/82–9/92."
144. Ibid.
145. Ibid.
146. Lisa Delorme, "The Ethics of Out-of-Country Midwifery Training," *Midwifery Matters*, Winter 2015, pp. 2–3.
147. https://midwivesofcolor.wordpress.com/2013/09/17/demand-for-ethical-midwifery-prompts-systemic-change-bastyr-university-department-of-midwifery-leads-the-way/.
148. Daily log, ND; (graduate is Beth Green), Coyote personal collection.
149. Beth Coyote, interview with author, July 25, 2015.
150. Jo Anne Myers-Cieck and Marcia Peterson, "Politics of Health Care," May 2, 1985 class lecture, 1 hour 45 min video, SMS archives.
151. Ina May Gaskin, "Interview with Jo Anne Myers-Ciecko," *Birth Gazette*, Summer 1997, Vol. 13 no. 3, p. 28, https://midwivesofcolor.wordpress.com/2013/09/17/demand-for-ethical-midwifery-prompts-systemic-change-bastyr-university-department-of-midwifery-leads-the-way/.
152. "SMS graduates," SMS Box 14.
153. "2010 grad speech" PowerPoint, Suzy Myers personal collection.
154. Ibid.
155. Myers, interview with author, July 21, 2015.
156. Myers, PowerPoint for ACNM conference, 2009.
157. http://bastyr.edu/academics/midwifery.

EPILOGUE

1. http://www.cedarbrooklodge.com/.
2. Saraswathi Vedam to Home Birth Summit Delegates, September 28, 2014, Home Birth Summit III Program, Wendy Kline personal collection.
3. https://www.huffingtonpost.com/entry/the-real-cost-of-giving-birth-in-the-us_us_5a144a83e4b05ec0ae8445d3.
4. https://www.propublica.org/article/severe-complications-for-women-during-childbirth-are-skyrocketing-and-could-often-be-prevented.
5. https://www.nytimes.com/2018/04/11/magazine/black-mothers-babies-death-maternal-mortality.html.
6. https://www.washingtonpost.com/news/wonk/wp/2014/09/29/our-infant-mortality-rate-is-a-national-embarrassment/?noredirect=on&utm_term=.891d8e8379ea.
7. http://www.homebirthsummit.org/summits/vision/statements/. Also printed in "Home Birth Summit III: Advancing Equity through Voice, Policy, Practice and Research," program, p. 5.
8. Home Birth Summit III Program, p. 6.
9. John Jennings, "Emergency Care Can Be Too Urgently Needed for Home Births," https://www.nytimes.com/roomfordebate/2015/02/24/is-home-birth-ever-a-safe-choice/emergency-care-can-be-too-urgently-needed-for-home-births.
10. Marinah Farrell, "Hospitals Carry Their Own Risks," https://www.nytimes.com/roomfordebate/2015/02/24/is-home-birth-ever-a-safe-choice/hospitals-carry-their-own-risks.
11. https://www.acog.org/-/media/Committee-Opinions/Committee-on-Obstetric-Practice/co697.pdf?dmc=1&ts=20170506T1034060833.
12. Home Birth Summit III Program, p. 18.
13. https://www.whynothome.com/directors-statement/.
14. Moore, "Why Not Home?" film transcript.

15. Ibid.

16. Jennie Joseph, "Why Not Home?" film transcript.

17. https://www.nytimes.com/2018/02/14/opinion/pregnancy-safer-women-color.html.

18. Ibid.

19. Saraswathi Vedam, "Why Not Home?" film transcript.

20. S. Vedam, K. Stoll, M. MacDorman, E. Declercq, R. Cramer, M. Cheyney, et al. (2018) "Mapping integration of midwives across the United States: Impact on access, equity, and outcomes," *PLoS ONE* 13(2): e0192523. https://doi.org/10.1371/journal.pone.0192523

21. Ibid.

22. Ibid.

23. https://www.nytimes.com/2018/04/11/magazine/black-mothers-babies-death-maternal-mortality.html.

24. https://www.nytimes.com/2018/04/20/opinion/childbirth-black-women-mortality.html.

25. https://www.propublica.org/article/midwives-study-maternal-neonatal-care.

26. Lester Hazell, "A Study of 300 Elective Home Births," *Birth and the Family Journal*, vol. 2 no. 1 (December 1974): 11–18.

INDEX